Recent Reforms in the Swedish Health Care System

Implications for the Swedish Welfare State

Randolph K. Quaye

UNIVERSITY PRESS OF AMERICA,® INC.
Lanham • Boulder • New York • Toronto • Plymouth, UK

Copyright © 2007 by
University Press of America,® Inc.
4501 Forbes Boulevard
Suite 200
Lanham, Maryland 20706
UPA Acquisitions Department (301) 459-3366

Estover Road
Plymouth PL6 7PY
United Kingdom

All rights reserved
Printed in the United States of America
British Library Cataloging in Publication Information Available

Library of Congress Control Number: 2007932475
ISBN-13: 978-0-7618-3788-6 (paperback : alk. paper)
ISBN-10: 0-7618-3788-4 (paperback : alk. paper)

Contents

Preface		v
Introduction		vii
1	The Swedish Health Care System in Focus	1
2	The State and the Medical Profession: Some Theoretical Concepts in Comparing Medical Professions Cross-Nationally	7
3	Managed Care and Doctoring in the United States	12
4	Health Care Market Systems and Reforms in Sweden	25
5	Diagnostic Related Groups (DRGs): Special Case of Reform in Sweden	36
6	Is the Swedish Welfare State in Retreat?: Current Trends in Swedish Health Care	48
7	Challenges for the Welfare States in Europe and the Way Forward	63
Appendix		67
Bibliography		73
Index		79

Preface

For the past decade, my research has focused on the changing status of the medical profession and the important role of the state in health care financing and delivery. My interest in the Swedish health care system goes back to the early1990s when I was awarded a faculty grant to Stockholm to conduct guided bibliographic research for a new course that I proposed and taught for pre-medicine students at Union College in Schenectady, New York. Little did I know that ten years later, I will be writing a book about the Swedish health care system.

Significantly, in recent years, economic incentives have become more and more important in health care, even in welfare countries such as Sweden where health care is primarily the responsibility of the state. In a decade and half, Sweden has experimented with different health care financing modalities. In Stockholm County, for example, the use of a performance-based reimbursement system has been studied and extensively discussed by Swedish scientists and scholars. So far as we know, relatively little research has been done on how these financial incentives over time have affected the views of physicians in Sweden. *Recent Reforms in the Swedish Health Care System* explores the impact of these financial incentives not only on the medical profession but the welfare state in Sweden in general.

Drawing upon current research, case studies, as well as recent works by the author on Sweden, I analyze the implications of these reforms on the future structure of the well-envied health care of Swedes. The manuscript appears at a timely moment, given the current debates on health care financing, and the wider implications of market forces on the quality, autonomy and delivery of health care cross-nationally.

My work was supported by the Ohio Wesleyan University TEW Presidential Discretionary Fund and the College of Wooster's Luce Fund for Distinguished

Scholarship. Chapter Three has appeared in slightly different form in the International Journal of Health Care Quality Assurance.

Chapter Four has appeared in a modified version in the European Journal of Public Health. I thank both editors for the permission to reprint these two articles.

My thanks are due to many people. Professor Stefan Hakansson of the Swedish National Board of Health and Welfare for graciously allowing me to use his office for my work. Helena Dahlgren for always taking time to talk to me. I certainly acknowledge the guidance and support from Martha Huggins, Malcolm Willison, Birgitta Danielsson, Ewa Forsberg, Goran Berleen, Annika Farrow, Ingemar Eckerlund , Goran Arrivdsson and Bength Linder. A special thanks to my father, Daniel Quaye, my brother, Daniel Quaye Jr, and my mother, Dora Bonney and aunt, Agnes Bonney. To Kwesi, Kofi, Kojo, Kobina, Asi, Asare Awuku, Mama Felicia and the larger family, this book is for you all. Thank you for all your support throughout the years.

Introduction

This book grew out of a decade of research on the changing status of the medical profession and the important role of the state in health care financing and delivery. For the past several years, I have been intrigued by the Swedish system of universal access to health, and by Swedes relatively general satisfaction with their health care system. At the same time, over the last decade or so, various forces have changed the thinking at several Swedish county councils and at the national level about how to control health care costs while simultaneously guaranteeing "good health and equal access to health services for everyone" (Swedish Association of Local Authorities and Regions, 2005). There is an increasing focus on, and concern about, the quality of medical care in Sweden.

Rising health care expenditures in all Western countries over the last two and half decades since 1980 have induced a "shift of impetus away from issues of access and affordability towards cost control" (Organization for Economic Cooperation and Development, 1995:49). In nearly all European countries, national governments initiated policies geared towards providing health care more efficiently through the introduction of market-oriented reforms. In Great Britain, it was widely believed that an alternative system could be devised that retained the advantages of the National Health Service while expanding consumer choice and reducing supply-side inefficiencies (OECD, 1995). This was to be achieved through the use of financial incentives such as diagnostic-related groups (DRGs) in health care.

Similarly, the Dekker Reform in the Netherlands and the Blum Reform in Germany focused on the introduction of market-oriented systems in the delivery of health care. For example, to address the problems of inefficiency and uncoordinated financing structures, the Dekker Reform of 1990 gave Dutch providers competitive incentives to produce cost-effective care and also streamlined the private insurance sector by creating a common risk-related insurance premium financed by the government in an attempt to eliminate the incentives for private insurance to dump costly patient to the exceptional medical expense scheme program. It also allowed the closing of the most inefficient hospitals and gave patients more health care choices (OECD, 1995; Quaye, 2001).

Under the Blum Reform, competition among German health care providers was encouraged through a diagnostic-related group (DRG)-based reimbursement payment system.

Sweden, despite its reduced health care expenditures in the 1990s, recognized the inefficiencies within its health system. In the last few years, discussions on the necessity of rationing care for cancer patients in Stockholm hospitals, and on the long waiting lists for hip replacement, cataract, and coronary surgery led many Swedish counties to initiate new ways of financing and organizing health care in Sweden (Hakansson, 1994). While extensive research has focused on the impact of financial incentives in the United States, very little is known about the impact of such cost control strategies on Swedish physicians' practice behavior. With a few notable exceptions, such as Hakansson (1994) and Forsberg (2001), most Swedish studies have focused on the effects of reforms on efficiency and productivity in health care delivery services. This study addresses a different and interesting topic, how physician behavior is affected by cost-control measures. In my earlier study, "Professional Integrity in the Age of Managed Care"(Quaye,2001), U. S. physicians in Ohio reported that managed care has robbed them of income, autonomy, and job satisfaction. Can such trends be observed in Sweden as well?

Significantly, in recent years, economic incentives have become more and more important in health care, even in countries such as Sweden where health care is regarded as the responsibility of the public sector. Approximately half of the county councils in Sweden have instituted a system of separate purchasers and providers, and performance-based reimbursements, measured according to diagnostic-related groups (DRGs) system. Several Swedish studies have shown that economic incentives do influence medical decision making (Neuhauser, 1987; Hillman et al., 1989; Hemenway et al., 1990; Forsberg, 2002).

Examining what is a much more public-financed system (90% of Swedish health budget is financed by the state) than exists in the United States provides a good contrast. After all, given the difference in philosophy between the Swedish state welfare state and a privately financed system such as in the United States, one might expect to see a different response to economic incentives among Swedish physicians compared with U. S. physicians. The exploration here of physician behavior in response to new payment methodologies (a system separating purchasers and providers, and performance-based reimbursement measured by a system of diagnostic-related groups) makes a new contribution to the field of health care studies because it allows exploration of the general pattern of emerging changes internationally in reimbursement strategies designed to alter physicians' behavior. Furthermore, this book has implications for investigating how these structural changes intersect with the particular design of the Swedish health care system and its politics in the light of the extensive reforms that were implemented there in the 1990s.

In an article by Cleary and Landon in the United States (1998:4), they reported that "Whereas physicians once practiced primarily alone or in small autonomous groups, they are now more likely to practice in large groups and are increasingly subjected to profiling, utilization review, and pre-approval for procedures and treatments." At the same time, they argued that, "'Physicians in the United States continue to enjoy higher salaries, more autonomy, and more prestige than in many countries." But with managed care, are doctors even in the United States experiencing what McKinlay and Stoeckle have called, the "de-professionalization" of the medical profession?

More generally, we are interested in the question of whether Western medicine is dying as a profession: Do physicians feel they are losing autonomy because of cost control strategies? Is this loss of control happening faster in some nations than others? How does the relationship between the state and the medical profession differ in the United States and Sweden? And where are physicians better off in terms of income, autonomy, and job satisfaction?

This book attempts to sketch changing trends in medical practice in both countries. The focus will be on Sweden with some specific references to the United States. My primary goal will be to explore the relationship between the Swedish state and the medical profession, particularly in an age of cost control and with the retreat of the welfare state in Sweden.

We will begin our discussion with a general introduction in Chapter One to the Swedish health care system. We conclude this chapter with a brief chapter summaries.

Chapter Two discusses the international literature on the varying state role in health care financing and regulation and assesses some theories on the impact of political and economic changes on the medical profession as well as reviewing the extensive literature on medical professionalism and the role of the state in the changing status of the medical profession.

Chapter Three discusses state interventions in U.S. health care financing and regulation through a study of Ohio physicians.

Chapter Four examines health care market reforms in Sweden in the early 1990s with a discussion on how these changes are affecting Swedish physicians.

Results of two surveys are presented. The impact of cost-control strategies on general practitioners, followed by a seven-year study assessing the role of internal market reforms on Swedish physicians' practice behavior is presented.

A contrast is offered with Sweden through an examination of the impact of managed care on U.S. physicians.

Chapter Five focuses on DRGs as a special issue in Swedish health care financing. Book explores the extensive discussion of the role of this reimbursement payment system on the delivery of care, and assess to what extent this payment system is undermining the Swedish goal of equal access to health care for all. The different experiences with the use of financial incentives in Swedish counties and the lessons to be learned from these market reforms in Sweden are discussed.

Chapter Six will examine current trends in Swedish health care.

Chapter Seven will discuss the health care challenges for the welfare states in Europe and examine the implications of these shifts for equity and access, and offer suggestions for future research.

Chapter One

The Swedish Health Care System in Focus

Health care in Sweden is regarded as an essential component of the welfare state. It is seen as a public good, and rooted in the solidarity principle of both vertical and horizontal equity. One of the fundamental principles is that all Swedes, irrespective of their income, age, race, or residence are guaranteed access to health care (Berleen, Hakansson, Rehnberg and Wennstrom, 1992). According to Mosher (1980:96), "The history of Sweden is filled with examples of how governments have shown tremendous sensitivity toward the maintenance and enhancement of the health of the population. The principles underlying this governmental attitude in Sweden are akin to those embedded in the concept of natural law." In this connection," The health care system is based on the concepts of shared need and collective responsibility rather than on the purchasing power of the individual" (Bjorkman,1985: 406). The introduction in 1955 of the compulsory social insurance entitled all Swedes to medical services. The planning of the welfare state was infused with the concept of social justice (jamlikhet), meaning all individuals have an equal right to live a rich and evolving life (Mosher, 1980:112).

While the system is highly centralized, the decision making about medical care is highly decentralized. Under the Health and Medical Services Act, "The county councils have the responsibility to provide health and medical services and to work for a good standard of health among the population"(Fact Sheet of Sweden, 1995). Twenty-three counties and the three municipal boroughs of Goteborg, Malmo, and Gotland are responsible for planning, financing and delivery of health care services (Bjorkman, 1985). According to the latest figures from Organization for Economic Co-operation and Development (OECD) 2005, the total Swedish expenditure on health as a percentage of Gross Domestic Product (GDP) was 8.4 percent compared to 13.5 percent in the United States. The sources for funding health care in Sweden are: proportional income taxes as well as indirect taxes, national social insurance system contributions, private insurance, and patient fees (European Observatory on Health Care Systems, 2001).

A fundamental aspect of the Swedish health care system is its regionalization. According to the Swedish Institute, regionalization in health care system refers to "The distribution and [regional] allocation of resources according to the types of care on three levels: primary or ambulatory, secondary or specialty care; and super-specialty services" (Mosher, 1980:119). The levels are linked which allows patients the opportunity to access all three. For example, the regional medical system operates at nine regional hospitals. There are sixty county/ district hospitals and eleven hundred health centers scattered throughout Sweden (Glenngard, Hjalte, Svensson, Anell and Bankkauskaite, 2004) According to the *Fact Sheet of Sweden* (1995), a relatively large proportion of the resources available for medical services have been allocated to the provision of care and treatment at the hospitals. That accounts for the high numbers of Swedes using the hospital as their primary access to care. In terms of administrative structure, under the Ministry of Health and Social Affairs is the National Board of Health and Welfare (socialstyrelsen), the Swedish Council of Technology Assessment in Health Care (statens) and the Medical Products Agency among others (see Figure 1.1 for details).

Another official body important for understanding the structure of the Swedish medical system is the Federation of County Councils now merged with the Local Authorities to form the Swedish Association of Local Authorities and Regions. The Council, according to Garpenby (1989:73), "could be characterized as a quasi-public organization. The association is funded out of public money and controlled by politicians having an electoral mandate from local [voters]. Its role is to represent the health care providers in discussions with central government and to negotiate terms of service with the health service unions."

The national government, through its exercise of financial control and regulation over the ability of county councils to impose taxes, has been able historically to determine the direction of the health care system. One clear example is the national government's moratorium on county councils imposing new taxes on the citizens in 1991.

Another earlier intervention by the national government in the early 1970s was the provisions under what became known as the Seven Crowns Reform. The reform "disallowed direct [financial] transactions between hospital physicians, who comprise the overwhelming majority of Swedish medical practitioners, and their patients" (Bjorkman, 1985:409). The reform, among other things, abolished the fee-for-service payment schedule for physicians and im-

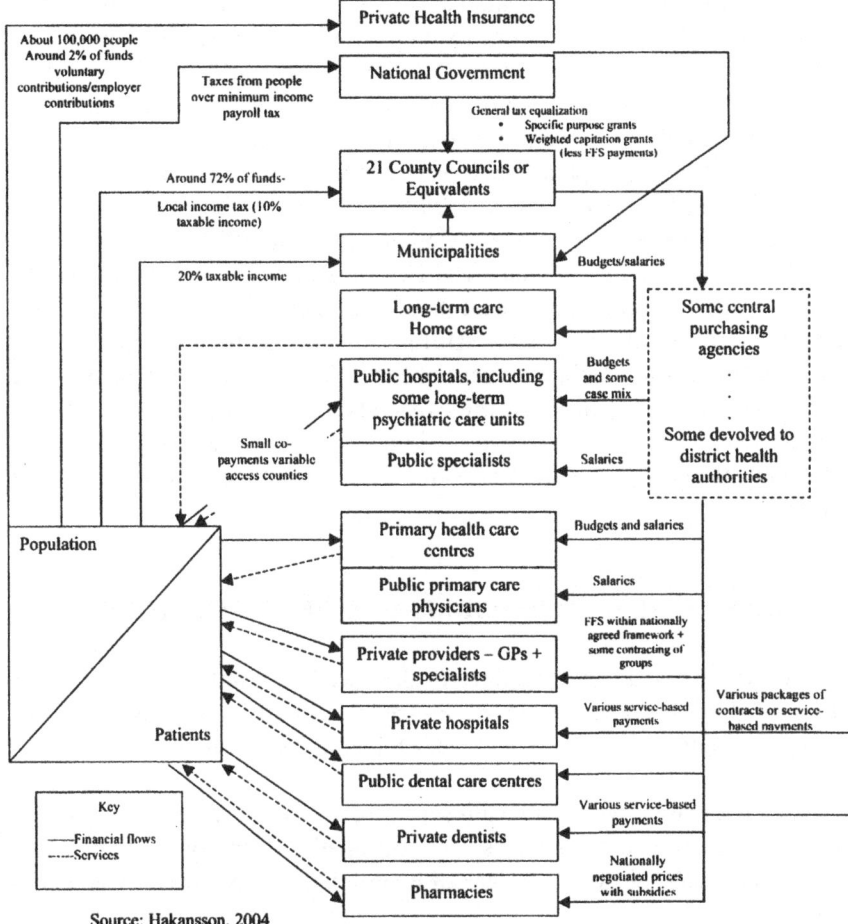

Figure 1.1. Sweden Health Care System Financing Flows 1999

posed a uniform fee for outpatient service. Under the reform, hospital physicians were put on regulated work schedules with fixed incomes (Hakansson and Nordling, 1997) thereby allowing the national government to not only control physicians' fees, but also health care costs.

In Sweden, less than 7 percent of health care practice has been private sector, even though as a result of recent changes, the proportion has increased to about 30 percent. As discussed by Hakansson and Nordling (1997), most physicians in Sweden work as salaried employees in primary care centers or hospitals. The hospital specialist, on average, earns about $35,400 Swedish crowns (SEK). While efforts have been made to strengthen access to primary care, this has not worked out because of the small number of trained general practitioners in the Swedish health care system. However, as a result of new reforms, the proportion of Swedes using the primary care services has increased from 42% in 1989 to 49% in 1990 (Hakansson & Nordling, 1997). In 2003, Sweden had eleven hundred health centers out of which three hundred were privately run. In addition, twenty-nine percent of all physician consultations in the total outpatient care were conducted at private facilities (Federation of Swedish County Councils, 2004). That the system has worked well until recently can be attested in a review by Saltman (1992). As he asserted, " Health care in Sweden, Finland, and Denmark is well-reputed for commitment to values of equity and social justice and health care systems in these three countries are the most successful in the industrialized world" (p.157). This reputation is no doubt the result of low infant mortality estimated to be about (four per 1000), and high life expectancy (78 years). But like all successful systems, there is still room for improvement and Sweden, like Great Britain and the other industrialized nations, is not immune from the challenge of reform.

ISSUES IN HEALTH REFORMS IN SWEDEN IN THE 1990S

In reviewing the main shortcomings of the Swedish health services, leading scholars led by (Ham, Robinson and Benzeval, 1990) have suggested the following as major issues facing the Swedish health care system:

- lack of integration between health services, social services, sickness benefits, early retirement, pensions, and occupational injury insurance and within the health sector itself, lack of integration between primary and hospital care;
- in the primary health care system, general practitioners do not act as "gatekeepers," resulting in a relatively high proportion of self-referrals by patients themselves to hospital outpatients and emergency departments;
- some regions experience difficulties in recruiting general practitioners;
- variations among individuals in health care utilization, which cannot be explained by differences in health problems;
- long waiting lists for some types of treatments, such as cataract, hip-joint and bypass surgery, although queues and lengths decreased in 2003 (Swedish Association of Local Authorities and Regions, 2005);
- patients sometimes have a limited choice, although improved in recent years;
- insufficient incentives for health personnel to improve productivity and efficiency, although improved in recent years (Swedish Association of Local Authorities and Regions, 2005).

Table 1.1. Swedish County Council Administrative Level Methods For Patient Care

County	Agency	Reimbursement Calculation
Bohus	County council	DRG—payment reduced if actual volume exceeds the plan
Dalarna	Purchasers	Mixed—cost ceilings and/or discounts, depending on purchaser
Stockholm	County council	DRG—payments reduced if actual volume exceeds the plan
Sormland	County council	Mixed-DRG—in several district areas payments reduced if actual volume exceeds the plan

Source: Anell, 1996:26

As a result of this confluence of forces, and a new Conservative majority's push for privatization and competition in health care in 1990, Sweden, like its other European counterparts, introduced several measures in an attempt to address the problems of inefficiency and limited choice for patients. As a result, several counties in Sweden introduced a purchaser-provider split in which county councils assumed the primary responsibility for purchasing services from health care providers, by instituting a system of reimbursement through the DRG system of payment. In this new regime, hospitals and physicians were paid according to patient outcomes, thereby allowing efficient providers to increase their productivity and guaranteeing efficiency and greater choice of physicians for patients. Table 1.1 summarizes the different payment models for somatic care in hospitals.

According to Bergman (1998:96) " two basic principles are common in all county councils: (1) the separation between purchaser and provider, having some sort of contract between them, and (2) the provider is paid by the district where the patient lives, money follows the patient and is related to a specific output or performance." For example, Table 1.2 shows counties that have instituted the purchaser-provider split.

Freedom in choice of providers is an essential aspect of the health care model in 11 out of 26 Swedish counties. Effective in 1992, the care guarantee, a maximum waiting time of three months for ten types of medical treatment, mostly

Table 1.2. Swedish County Councils and Purchaser Organizations

County Councils	Purchaser Organization
Bohus	14 purchasers, based on former primary care districts
Dalarna	15 purchasers, based on former primary care districts
Stockholm	9 purchasers, based on former health care districts
Somland	1 purchaser, based on former central administration

Source: Anell, 1996:24

surgical, was introduced in all county councils (Anell, 1996). This allows patients to seek care outside their counties if it cannot be obtained within three months in their own county. The county in which the patient resides is obliged to pay the county providing the service. This, no doubt, has had an influence on hospital productivity and a reduced queue for elective surgeries, a phenomenon which had been endemic in the Swedish health care delivery system.

The Liberal–Conservative majority in parliament in 1993 introduced Proposition 1992/93:160 aptly referred to as the "house doctor scheme (Bergman,1998). The house doctor scheme had as its goal the encouraging of privatization among primary care physicians. For example, Section 5 of the Act allowed family doctors to keep a special list of the patients they serve, and the remuneration paid to these doctors consisted of a fixed amount of money for each case (capitation). The goal was to reduce the use of hospital resources by strengthening the primary care sector (Quaye, 2001). This legislation was repealed by the Social Democrats who returned to power in 1994, even though aspects of the provision have been retained by some other county councils.

In 1992, the Adel Reform was introduced. This was a program designed to reform care for the elderly. The reforms transferred responsibility for their care from county councils to local municipalities. Under this reform municipalities were given the responsibility for establishing special residential forms of service and care for those needing it. It is also the duty of the municipalities to operate assistance and medical services in the special housing for the elderly. Municipalities also incur the financial costs of acute medical and geriatric care (Federation of Swedish County Council, 1993). The implication of these reforms on the perspectives of Swedish physicians is explored in Chapter 6.

In summary, then, as Saltman (1993: 163) accurately describes it, "Current movement toward planned market models in the Nordic countries, although impressive in design, has yet to be fully tested in application[and] the extent to which the pursuit of heightened efficiency and performance is compatible with continued maintenance of social values like equity and comprehensiveness remains to be seen." I will return to these issues but for now will turn our attention to a more extensive discussion of the Swedish state's role in health care and of the status of the medical profession within that context.

Chapter Two

The State and the Medical Profession: Some Theoretical Concepts in Comparing Medical Professions Cross-Nationally

This chapter considers the literature on the relationship between the state, the medical profession, and consumers, and assess the extent to which these relationships seem to undermine the power and autonomy of Swedish physicians. In particular, I will examine the impact of recent financial incentives on the practice and quality of Swedish health care services. We will explore whether the socialization of physicians is changing because of the need to control health care cost. What lessons can be learned from the Stockholm Model and are the results likely to be duplicated elsewhere in Sweden? Why is the gate keeping role of primary care physicians not developed as in the English system, for example? What role do politics play in the Swedish health care system? To what extent are the state, the profession, and even capitalism involved in a full welfare state? How have developments in terms of cost-control measures in the 1990s affected the nature of the relations among actors? What are the directions of gain or loss in the influence of parties (Social Democrats) on the left and on the right (Center Right) in health care management? As might be expected, leftist parties in Sweden have historically been against fee-for service. Conversely, parties of the Right favor a retreat by the welfare state and a greater privatization in the health care sector. What is the history of the Swedish Medical Association in protecting its member's interests against assault by the welfare state? And how has the role of the state evolved in Sweden?

But before I attempt to answer these questions, I will briefly discuss four key terms: (i) "profession", (ii) "state", (iii) "corporatism" and (iv) "deprofessionalization".

PROFESSIONS

According to Krause (1996), the term "profession" is used to describe an occupation in which members have control over their work because of the extensive training and expertise of its members. In medicine, this depends not only many years of medical training, but the fact that the authority of the physician is conferred through the licensing process by physician's professional association itself and confirmed by the state. Members of the profession uphold their code of ethics, and they are self-governing as members of their own professional association and subjected to some measure of peer control. Ultimately under this model, members have autonomy in their work.

STATE

The state is central to any discussion of the status of the medical profession. For this reason, we define the state by adopting the definition used by Krause. Krause defines states as "bodies that possess a monopoly over the means of force, as well as most of the means of sustaining the society through education and professional training" (Krause, 1996: 22). Frenk and Duran–Arenas (1993:27) define the state as "the institution of government, providing the administrative, legislative, and judicial vehicles for the actual exercise of public authority and power rather than the broad definition of the state as the total political organization of a society." Frenk and Duran-Arenas argue that for Weber, "Bureaucracy and professionalization are two expressions of a single process of increased rationalization in western societies." Parsons extends this concept by isolating two ideas of authority: The first is based on the "authority of the office" rooted in a rational legal organizational structure, and the second, on the authority of expertise which characterizes professional work (p.30). Friedson would argue that in situations where the profession has autonomy and self-regulates, the professionals dominate the definition of their role in the larger socio-political system. On the other hand, McKinlay and Haug would argue that given the controls exerted by the state bureaucracy, the power of the professionals is ultimately circumscribe by bureaucracy—in the case of medicine, both the state and the private corporations such as insurance companies. Further, Weber defines the state as the organization whose essential characteristics is its monopoly of the legitimate use of physical force (Weber, 1946b:78). In this way, the state creates the structures possible for professional associations to gain practice monopoly and thereby control their members' professional work. As a result, the state and private bureaucracies can intervene to mediate the relationship between providers and clients.

In Sweden, state power has been legislated through the Swedish Medical Services Act in which the state set the broader goals for the nation by guaranteeing equal access to health care for all Swedes. The state also through its financing structures has worked hard historically to maintain two principles: (1) The solidarity principle, in which the poor and the elderly are guaranteed access to health care irrespective of income and age, and(2)the equity principle which guarantees contributions from all citizens based on ability to pay. In a nutshell, the exercise of state power in health care, according to Frenk and Duran-Arenas (1993) can be traced to four areas: penetration, standardization, participation, and redistribution.

Scholars have drawn a distinction between state centralization and state pluralism. According to Garpenby (1989), state centralism exists where various groups interests are merged under one state authority (e.g. Communist Party). State pluralism, on the other hand exists where the state plays a more limited role allowing different corporatist organizations to function and different competing interest groups to struggle for power and control.

The USA health care system is a classic example of state pluralism—where health care organizations, health insurance companies, health product industries, professional associations, labor unions and other interest groups struggle for control.

On the other hand, Sweden, like Germany, has a system of state centralization in which the national federal government lays down and enforces basic rules within which strong regional governments exercise control over economic and health activities through their well-developed councils and municipalities.

It has been assumed that in "high-stateness" nations, professions have little power because they cannot organize themselves as private autonomous groups (Friedson,1970:58). The assumption is rooted in the claim that, since medical professions in such societies have no formal association, independent of the state, and state agencies are responsible for legitimizing and directing their affairs, they lack power to influence state policy on how doctors are trained, nor on their income, prestige and working conditions.

These characteristics may accurately reflect the Swedish experience. For example, the delayed organization of the Swedish Medical Association prevented it from influencing legislation passed to regulate the medical market. The Swedish medical profession in the 1960s cooperated with the state through the National Board of Health and Welfare which granted the profession its privileges (Garpenby,1989:48).

Another Swedish example of state intervention in health care was the 1969 Seven Crowns Reform. This reform established a fee schedule for hospital stays and turned most physicians unto salaried employees responsible for both inpatient and outpatient care, with no rights to place private patients in public hospitals. The reform also increased admission to state medical schools, leading to an over-supply of doctors. This was followed in 1984 by the Dagmar Reform, aimed at curbing the increase in private physicians by requiring physicians who wanted to establish their own private practice to apply for permission from the local government (Garpenby, 1989). More recent state interventions will be examined in later chapters.

CORPORATISM

By corporatism we mean a condition where interest groups in civil society are able to influence the state. For example, trade unions. The Swedish medical profession has become moderately powerful since it is now strong enough to deal with other equally organized bodies of civil society. The Swedish Medical Association, which includes 92% of physicians as members strongly supports a trade union philosophy and has spoken out in support of physicians on health policy issues (Garpenby, 1989).

DEPROFESSIONALIZATION

Paul Starr had predicted that "the last decades of the twentieth century are likely to be a time of diminishing resources and autonomy for many physicians" (Starr,1982:421). Most scholars had never envisage, that medicine would experience a transformation of such great proportions and that the "dominant profession" as Friedson (1970) described it, would experience increased pressures in the delivery of health care services as a result of the growth of managed care. Approximately, eighty-five percent of all insured employees in the United States have moved out of traditional fee-for-service into managed care plans (Iglehart, 1999). The growth of managed care has led several scholars to conclude that medicine has lost its status as a dominant profession (Haug,1977; McKinlay and Stoeckle, 1989). This is particularly true as managed care imposes financial incentives, restrictions on offered care, and gag clauses which undermine the patient-doctor relationship (Shortell, 1989; Quaye, 2001). According to Stephen O'Connor and Joyce Lanning (1992), the challenge to American physicians self-determination are both direct and indirect. They draw attention to demands from third-party providers, the need for prior authorization for needed services, the Medicare prospective-payment system and state and national regulations as forces undermining the autonomy of physicians. Haug, assessing the impact of these changes on U. S. doctoring, argues that "Medicine has been losing its prestigious societal position and the trust that goes with it" (p.83) She argues that autonomy from exclusive control of medical knowledge has been compromised and corrupted by the growth of physicians technology and the availability of doctors on line. She attributes some of these changes to the impact of managed care and the demystification of medicine brought about by wider education, knowledge, and the growth of health clubs hence the term "deprofessionalization". Wolinsky (1988) suggests further that rather than 'deprofesionalization" bringing about the end of professional dominance, "corporatization" will transform the context in which the profession is dominant." This certainly is the case, given the growth of managed care and its impact on physicians' professional behavior. Using a Marxian framework, McKinlay and Stoeckle assert that, " The growing corporatization and bureaucratization of medicine have resulted in eliminating the self-employment and autonomy of physicians" (p.115). They point to several assaults on the profession through state regulations such as anti-dumping legislation and growth of physician assistants and non-clinical physicians etc.

The wider implications of the changes in physicians' sources of income for the status of the medical profession is compared in this work cross nationally also in this chapter by examining the perspectives of U. S. physicians in active practice in the state of Ohio. The comparison to Swedish physicians is illustrative for after all physicians in the United States continue to enjoy higher salaries, more autonomy, and more prestige than their Swedish counterparts. What has not been fully explored so far, however, is the state role in health care and the medical socialization experienced by both American and Swedish physicians, which this chapter will introduce.

Chapter Three

Managed Care and Doctoring in the United States

This chapter reports on a study conducted among physicians in Ohio on the impact of managed care on their professional practice.

By 1998, approximately eighty-five percent of all insured employees in the United States had moved out of traditional fee-for-service plans into managed care plans (Iglehart, 1999). The number of Americans receiving their health care through employer-sponsored health maintenance organizations rose from 15 million in 1988 to 50 million in 1996 (Bodenheimer, 1998). At the same time, the percentage of physicians with managed care contracts increased from 61 percent to 75 percent (Warren, Weitz and Kulis, 1999). Recent studies on the impact of managed care on American physicians have focused on states with high managed-care penetration and where bonuses have been used extensively as financial incentives to restrict care. But there has been relatively little research on physicians practicing in smaller communities and towns.

In their study on the views of managed care, Simon et al. (1999) focused broadly on the views of students, residents, faculty, and deans at medical schools. While the impact of managed care has been widely debated and researched, few studies have focused on ordinary practicing physicians' views and relatively little on how these changes have affected career aspirations in the profession as a whole. In this chapter we report on the views of physicians about the impact of managed care on their professional practice.

BACKGROUND

"Managed care" refers to health maintenance organizations and preferred provider organizations that "manage or control the cost of health care" (Steinberg,1997). Freeborn and Pope (1994:6) define managed care as the "control of access to, and limitations on, physician and patient utilization of services by public or private payers or their agents through the use of prior and concurrent review for approval of services and financial incentives or penalties." Cost-containment measures such as managed care have slowed increases in U.S. health care expenditure. It is estimated that managed care saved between US $150 billion to US $250 billion in 1997 year alone out of a total United States health spending of one trillion dollars (MacDonald, 1998). At the same time, Time/CNN poll reported that three-fourths of HMO members were satisfied with their health care (MacDonald, 1998). But what about physicians, who until recently were seen to be advocates for their patients? As Shortell (1998) noted, " A physician in a managed care organization cannot be an unrestricted advocate of each patients' best interest." Herein lies the dilemma.

In his article, " Physicians Seek Remedy: Doctors Battle HMO," Marquis (1999:B1) asserts that "Doctors are complaining that the era of managed care has robbed them of autonomy, quality, income, time, prestige—even respect." Our next discussion reports on the perspectives of physicians in northeastern Ohio.

METHODS

These research data come from a survey mailed to physicians randomly selected from the Cigna Directory of Physicians practicing in Ohio. The questionnaires were developed on the basis of a systematic review of the literature on managed care. Since managed care operates largely on expense capitation and on financial incentive to keep down costs, and since the growth of managed care is a recent phenomenon, I wanted to explore the relationship of age, gender, type of specialty, financial incentive on their job satisfaction and other aspects of their situation. Given the divergent views of what managed care is, we purposely asked our respondents to describe what they understood "managed care" to mean. To ensure a high response rate, we included a stamped self-addressed envelope with the mailed questionnaire (See Appendix for Questionnaire).

The subjects were asked their specialty, total years of practice, practice conditions, and what percentage of their practice is HMO-based. Questions also focused on whether their arrangements with managed care included some type of financial incentive in the form of a bonus. They were also asked (on a Likert scale from 1= strongly disagree to 5= strongly agree) on whether they feel pressured by HMOs to limit referrals and whether they feel such pressures compromise patients' care.

The questionnaires were sent by regular mail between March and June of 1999 to a random sample of 150 licensed physicians in active practice in the cities of Akron, Cleveland, Wooster, and Canton in northeastern Ohio. Twelve individuals were eliminated from the sample because they could not be reached (the letters were returned indicating they were no longer at their old address and had left no forwarding addresses). The response rate was 51.3 percent.

RESULTS

Of the survey respondents, 92 percent were male, 7 percent were female; 31 percent were primary care physicians and 69 percent were specialists. Overwhelmingly, 98 percent of our respondents reported that they participated in at least some form of managed care. A total of 25 percent reported that 10 percent or less of their practice was HMO-based, 30 percent reported between 11 to20 percent, 16 percent reported 21–30 percent. About 29 percent reported that 31 percent or more of their practice was HMO-based. Half of our respondents reported that the net income from their practice was between $110,000 and $210,000, with most of the other half earning between $160,000 and $210,000 a year.

PHYSICIANS' VIEW ON THE MEANING OF MANAGED CARE

When respondents were asked to explain what "managed care" meant, many defined managed care as a cost-control measure, third party payers determining the appropriate level of care for an individual.

Most stressed that it meant physicians were "double agents" who must serve both patients and the organizations that pay for their care. As one respondent put it, "Managed care has taken away my ability to control my fees. It has taken away my ability to prescribe medicine and it has greatly increased my office overhead due to increased administrative work and increased the hassles in my job that do not improve patient care."

After all, the purpose of managed care is to improve the "bottom line" of the insurance company or managed care corporations. A physician stated that, " I do not know what 'managed care' really means. As practiced today, managed care equals managed health care." A 55-year old pathologist with 20 years of practice defined "managed care" as "insurance companies practicing medicine without a license, that is, payers determining the appropriate level of care for an individual patient without any medical training and no knowledge of the individual patient's status. Medicine cannot be practiced in cookbook fashion." An obstetrician with 5 years of practice defined managed care as " more paper work, phone calls for authorization, denial of necessary procedures, and fighting for patients' rights and against decreased reimbursement."

From the perspective of one physician, managed care means "medical care at reduced cost to the employer who pays for the insurance. It is cost containment to the provider, profit to the insurance industry and fairly reasonable quality of care." Another physician wrote that it often gets in the way between the physician and the patient's best medical interest.

As one cardiologist put it, " The concept of managed care is fundamentally sound, [but] Its implementation is arbitrary and capricious. Providers' input is non-existent. The absence of standardization makes it confusing to both providers and patients."

Given these kinds of criticism, not surprisingly, 97 percent of the respondents were opposed to managed care. But it is important to mention also that in our sample only 8 percent of the respondents reported that their arrangement with managed care also included some type of financial incentive for limiting patients' health care.

CLINICAL DECISION MAKING AND EXPERIENCES WITH CARE

When asked if they felt pressure from HMOs to limit referrals, 34 percent reported that they felt pressured and 18 percent reported that such pressures compromised care. About 31 percent reported that they felt some pressure to see more patients daily. Thirty-nine percent reported that pressures to see more patients compromised patient's care.

When respondents were asked to discuss what they perceived to be the impact of managed care on patients, they overwhelmingly mentioned that managed care limited the choice of both physicians and patients. One respondent declared:

> Managed care has left most patients bewildered as to what is and is not covered. It has made patients more tentative to accept treatment, not because of concern about the merits of the recommended therapy, but because of uncertainty of whether or not their carrier will agree.

Another announced that "The patient is short-changed. They are rushed in and out of doctors and the hospital in a manner that is inconsistent with quality care. Our system is failing fast and the insurance company is profiting."

Another stated, "The doctor-patient contract is automatically violated in care." Finally, from the perspective of another physician, the impact of managed care is "the loss of the patients' control of their bodies and souls to the company store."

EFFECTS OF MANAGED CARE ON PROFESSIONAL AUTONOMY

When respondents were asked if doctors are losing autonomy under managed-care systems, 97 percent stated that doctors are losing control. They reported that their income had decreased and that job security had deteriorated. In the words of a surgeon, "Anytime some one else dictates one's income and one's treatment regimen one has lost autonomy." Another stated that there "are many decisions made by people with no expertise and no understanding of the individual's problem. It is purely based on the bottom line, not quality."

A family physician echoed this sentiment when he stated that " I spend two hours a week attending meetings on how to cut costs to keep the hospital viable. You are treated like an employee who either complies or has your contract cancelled."

Another hospital physician noted that, "This is a needless question. I do not set my fees. I am told how quickly to see patients, what tests I should or should not order, what drugs I can prescribe, where I can refer and admit patients. I work harder and harder with more frustration and my income has not changed in ten years."

Another stated that, "We are now just employees with no labor rights due to federal anti-trust laws."

The majority of the respondents reported that managed care has significantly diminished their autonomy. The response by one family physician sums it up:

> Health care is a partnership among providers, patients, and carriers. For the most part, the patient-provider relationship is good, but the relationship with the carrier is pathetic. The ability to refer a patient to the best referral, is many times limited by managed care contracts; fighting for the patient's right to get the best care is exhausting, time-consuming, and interferes with the physician time with the patient. I believe this affects the quality of care as well as the physician's autonomy. Income reduction is now starting to force physicians to provide services that are less personal and labor-intensive.

SATISFACTION

However, when physicians were asked if they were satisfied with their work, two-thirds reported that they were generally satisfied. Only 18 percent reported that they were not. We also observed that those physicians who are largely involved in managed care were more likely to report that they were less satisfied with their work. This finding is consistent with other research findings (Warren et al., 1998, 1999; Simon et al., 1999). When this question was explored further by asking the respondents if they would highly recommend the medical profession to their children and /or relatives, about half (50.7 %) reported that they were less likely to do so. This raises an interesting paradox. Perhaps our respondents were reacting more to perceived future trends within medicine as they relate to work schedules and income. But from this survey, we do not have any way of knowing.

DISCUSSION

This chapter has covered Ohio physicians on the effects of managed health care on their medical practice. The results of the study suggest that managed care has had a negative impact on how they practice medicine. Several of our respondents reported that they are double agent and feel a strong sense of frustration. The degree of antipathy towards managed care differs between primary care physicians and specialists. As expected, primary care physicians were more likely to see their autonomy greatly diminished by the penetration of managed-care plans. The most interesting aspect of our finding is the reluctance of physicians, especially of primary care physicians not to recommend the profession to immediate family members. While it is difficult to draw precise conclusions from their responses, it seems quite likely that they are reacting to the continued growth of managed care and what they see as its negative influence in changing their work conditions.

While this study did not specifically address the effects of financial incentives on the quality of care (given the small percentage of the respondents, only 9 percent who responded to that part of the question in the survey), the fact that 41 percent reported that they were under pressure to see more patients and to limit referrals speaks to a broader issue within managed health care. Our study has confirmed previous studies about the negative consequences of managed care on both physicians and patients (Melden,1994; Steinberg,1997).

According to Marquis, "The growing prevalence of HMOs has clearly left a large [number] of the nation's health care providers disgruntled—a situation that can only damage the quality of care received by patients" (Marquis,1999.3). That 87 percent of our respondents support the right of patients to sue their HMOs is further testimony to the loss of autonomy by physicians in the delivery of health care.

It is clear that HMOs affect the delivery of health care in several ways. The emphasis on cost-containment negatively affects physicians' attitudes towards patient care and encourages the hiring of less-trained individuals as health care providers. Indeed, it can lead to rationing of health care (Steinberg, 1997).

To reduce the degree of frustration reported by our respondents, it is necessary for states, insurance companies, employers, patients, and physicians to establish channels of communication that could help alleviate some of the physicians' concerns and other critics. A medical health care board, similar to the Swedish Medical Board of Health and Welfare could provide a clearinghouse for dissemination of medical and insurance information to the general public.

Managed care is here to stay in the United States, but the financial losses incurred by Kaiser Permanante and other managed-care plans, as well as increased health care costs, appear to threaten the confidence of employers that managed care is the answer. The reality, though, is that U. S. employers are going to look for cost-efficient ways to provide health care for their employees, and managed-care organizations have been consistently proven to provide health care at lower cost. In the meantime, unless current trends change, we are likely to see other U.S. states follow the leadership of such states as California, Texas, and Georgia in approving versions of the Patient Bill of Rights. The recent bi-partisan congressional approval for the HMO bill of rights is a case in point.

This study is limited by small sample size and our reliance only on practicing physicians. A broader approach, incorporating the experience of patients and administrators of managed-care organizations would provide a broader understanding of the role of managed care in the U.S. health delivery system. Nevertheless, since physicians' activities constitute 70 percent of the cost in health care, understanding how they feel about managed care is critically important. It must also be added that since we let the respondents define managed care for themselves, it is possible that their responses may be limited only to their own experience and not necessarily about the overall effects of penetration of managed care more generally in the United States.

To further assess the impact of managed care on physicians, a follow-up study was conducted between April and June 2002. This time the sample was drawn from the 2001 American Medical Association Physician Masterfile for the state of Ohio. In addition, a diverse pool of minority and foreign-trained physician was purposively sampled from the list. Questionnaires were mailed to a total of 100 licensed physicians.

The key items identified in the questionnaire were:

- personal and demographic characteristics: age, gender race/ ethnicity (white, African American, Hispanic American, American Indian, Asian American and other), total years of practice;

- professional characteristics: medical fields, percentage of income based on fee for service and on managed care; their percentage of HMO-based practice; whether they have any arrangement with managed care that includes some type of financial incentive. For example, for cost-cutting in the form of bonuses.
- location of training and practice: the state or country where they trained, location of residency training. Factors that influenced their decision to become physicians.
- practice experience: We classified communities of practice as rural, urban or inner city, and explored whether they were likely to be practicing in states or counties where they had fulfilled their medical residency requirements.
- perspective on medical profession as a career: Whether they are satisfied with their practice and will recommend the profession to their relatives and/or children.
- whether they felt a diminished level of job security because of current changes in U.S. health care and whether their medical training prepare them well for current practice dealing with managed care systems.
- perspectives on quality of care.

ANALYSIS

Frequency distributions were obtained using the SPSS statistical package for all the variables. Data were assumed to be representative of the targeted population of physicians. Person's product correlation coefficient with statistical significance (p.values up to .20) were analyzed. The small sample size precluded further cross tabulation of the data.

RESULTS

Of the total of 100 questionnaires mailed, 50 were returned (an overall response rate of 50%). Most of the respondents were male (90%). About sixty-six of the respondents were in the age category of 46 to 65 years. Eighty-four percent of the sample reported practicing medicine for more than 10 years. As outlined in Table 3.1, 46 percent of the sample were primary/family care physicians and 54 percent were specialists in surgery, pediatrics, oncology or cardiology. Sixty-two percent reported that their income was derived from fee-for-service, while 26 percent attributed it to capitation by managed-care organizations. This would seem to suggest that

Table 3.1. Demographic and Professional Characteristics of Physician Respondents

Gender	Number	Percent (%)
Male	45	90
Female	5	10
Total	50	100

Age		
25–35	6	12
36–45	9	18
46–55	21	42
56–65	12	24
66+	2	4
Total	50	100

Payment Mode		
Fee for service	31	62
HMO	13	26
N/A	6	12
Total	50	100

Years of Practice		
1–5	2	4
6–10	6	12
11–15	9	18
16–20	10	20
21+	23	46
Total	50	100

Percentage of Practice HMO-based		
1–10	21	42
11–20	11	22
21–30	7	14
31–40	4	8
41–51	2	4
52+	0	0
N/A	5	10
Total	50	100

Medical Field		
Primary Care Physician	23	46
Specialist	27	54
Total	50	100

Race/Ethnicity		
White	35	70
Asian (India)	7	14
Hispanic	5	10
Native American	1	2
African-American	0	0
Other	2	4
Total	50	100

Urban/Rural Practices Location		
Rural	36	72
Urban America	10	20
Inner City	4	8
Total	50	100

the bulk of physicians still depend on fee-for-service systems of payment. What was unexpected was the low number of physicians (6 %) who reported that at least, thirty percent of their practice was based on health maintenance organizations. Whereas 42 percent reported that up to 10 percent of their practice was HMO based; Twenty-two percent reported that 11 to 20 percent was based on HMO, followed by 14 percent of that (21–30%) payment were HMO-based. Almost three fourths worked in non inner city urban areas. This was followed by 20 percent who reported practicing in rural areas and 8 percent in inner cities.

I was also interested in exploring if there was any relationship between location of residency training and eventual medical practice. In a study by Burfield et al. (1986), the authors observed a strong geographic relationship between training and practice. I wanted to assess whether this was consistent with our earlier study. From the analysis, 40 percent of the physicians trained in a particular state ended up practicing there after their residency supporting Burfield's earlier study about the importance of medical education training programs as gateways for attracting and recruiting physicians to practice in particular areas. I explored factors that influenced the decision of physicians to practice medicine in the first place. This study confirmed that one of the single most important reasons among multiple responses by respondents for why they entered the medical profession was to serve people (76%), followed by income (40%). Family tradition and prestige tied as the third reason (34%) and 20 percent offered other reasons. When the respondents were asked to indicate on a Likert scale of "very important" to "least important" factors that influenced their decision to practice in a specific region, family consideration were mentioned as the most important factor by 52 percent of the respondents. It was followed by availability of resources by 38 percent, access to professional colleagues by 30 percent and income by 22 percent.

Since several of the respondents were working under both retrospective fee-for-service payment and prospective payment systems (capitation), I wanted to examine their views on the effect of these payment methods on quality of care and service delivery. To investigate this, I asked the respondents to evaluate what type of payment system offers the best outcome for patients under different treatment models. Table 3.2 summarizes the results. Overwhelmingly, the respondents reported that the fee-for-service payment model is superior to managed care on all indicators measured.

In addition, I was interested in exploring if their age has influenced physicians' choice of specialty. Given the growing discussion on the negative effects of managed care on the practice of medicine, as well as the greater degree of antipathy toward managed care among primary care physicians, especially those who are younger, I explored whether the sample felt that younger physicians, were more likely to choose primary care as their choice of practice. The

Table 3.2. Result of Payment Methods on Quality Of Care (Ohio, 2002)

Service Delivery Model	Payment Method (%)		
	FFS	MC	NA
Better management of chronic illness	54	30	16
Better quality of end of life	62	24	14
Better continuity of care	70	18	12
Easier access to one's physician	92	2	6
Better referral service	92	2	6
Autonomy of work	94	0	6

sample question was, "Are younger physicians more likely to specialize in primary care than older physicians?" Using the schematic approach by Cohen et al.(1990), we classified young physicians as those under age 45 who had been in practice for more than one year but fewer than six years. There were not observable perceived differences among the respondents between age and choice of practice as well as differences between fee-for-service and capitated physicians.

PERSPECTIVES ON THE MEDICAL PROFESSION

However, to gauge more closely the career satisfaction of physicians, they were asked, "Given what you know about medicine as a profession, will you recommend this profession to your children or relatives?" This was measured on a Likert scale of "strongly agree" to "not at all."

More than half (56%) reported "not at all." These findings confirm earlier studies about increasing disenchantment with the practice of medicine at least from the perspective of our sample.

Physicians were asked if they were satisfied with their own medical practice. On this question, 78 percent reported that they were personally satisfied with their work. About 20 percent of the sample reported that they were less than fully satisfied with their work.

To explore the relationship between degree of satisfaction with years of practice, I examined this relationship. The findings suggest that older physicians (56–65 year of age) expressed greater dissatisfaction over their work. The chi square was 16.20 and the p. value was .01. The same trend was observed when physicians were asked whether they would recommend the profession to their children or relatives. The chi square was 11.08 and the p. value was .01 with a greater proportion of older physicians (33%) reporting "less likely to recommend" than younger physicians (16%).

QUALITY OF CARE

Physicians were asked whether they were concerned that the quality of care had declined for their patients in the previous two years. About two-thirds (70%) reported that they were very concerned about declining quality of care. There were no significant differences by age. Overwhelmingly, all physicians, regardless of age or specialty, were pessimistic about the future of health care in the United States.

TRAINING IN DEALING WITH MANAGED CARE

The respondents were asked whether medical school training prepared them well also in their current practice in dealing with managed care. The majority of the respondents (74%) indicated emphatically that they were not equipped to deal with managed care. The respondents reported that they felt a diminished level of job security because of current changes in health care.

About half of the respondents reported that they see on the average, 50–150 patients per week. It is important to note that those more involved with managed care than those less involved reported less job security (46%). Years of practice were correlated with job satisfaction. The b. coefficient was (34.74), suggesting that about 34 percent of the variance toward dissatisfaction was due to years of practice. A similar correlation between type of specialty and the likelihood of recommending the medical profession to children or relatives was also found.

DISCUSSION

The findings have confirmed that there is a strong relationship between region of residency training and location of practice after graduation. Second, physicians are worried about the diminishing quality of care for their patients in the face of cost-control measures. Third, older physicians are more likely to voice dissatisfaction with care and less likely to recommend the medical profession to their immediate family or relatives. There is a feeling of job insecurity experienced by those surveyed. Primary care physicians reported greater loss of autonomy than specialists did.

Overwhelmingly, physicians selected the fee-for-service payment method over capitation. But given the increased penetration of managed care, they may not have much leeway but will have to succumb to capitation as a predominant form of payment. Family considerations were mentioned as the single most important factor influencing the location of medical practice. In my original research I had wanted to explore the extent to which race and gender impacts on choice of practice and attitudes toward working conditions. I was interested in investigating if the experience of overwhelmingly whites physicians reported in the literature would be different from the experience of women and racial minorities in America. But the non-representation of women and of African Americans and the heavy predominance of white male physicians made this impossible. From the study, satisfaction and career aspirations of physicians were negatively related to age, number of years of practice, and capitation payment methods.

This study had several drawbacks. First was the low response rate. This made it difficult to explore the importance of gender and race in understanding the perspectives of Ohio physicians.

Second, what was meant by "job satisfaction" was not defined for the respondents and therefore their responses are likely to reflect more on their specific working conditions than their own satisfaction with being a physician.

Nevertheless, the views of physicians on their job experience could be assessed. Understanding how physicians feel about their practice and career aspirations are important and have major implications for patient care. After all, a satisfied physician is more likely to deliver better quality care for patients. As we better understand the changing role of health care financing in the United States, understanding how physicians see these changes in the light of their work is very important for the future of medicine in the United States.

The discussion so far suggests that managed care in the United States has seriously affected the professional autonomy and satisfaction of physicians. While these changes are monumental, I am not inclined to say that we are faced with the death of the medical profession in the United States. One can agree with Krause and Friedson that medicine as we knew it is gone and that state regulation and increased consumer demands are revolutionizing the practice of medicine in the United States. But the question is whether these changes are occurring in other countries as well, particularly in Sweden, a welfare state, where health care financing has been a function of the public sector. Are Swedish physicians experiencing the same changes as a result of the introduction of cost control measures? What follows, examines the impact of recent market reforms on doctoring in Sweden.

Chapter Four

Health Care Market Systems and Reforms in Sweden

Sweden, despite its reduced health care expenditures in the 1990s, recognized the inefficiencies within its system. Discussions on the necessity of rationing care for cancer patients in Stockholm hospitals and the long waiting lists for hip replacement, cataract, and coronary surgery led many Swedish county councils to initiate new ways of financing and organizing health care in Sweden (Hakansson, 1994). Reforms introduced in Sweden included, maximum guaranteed waiting times setting by the Federation of County Councils in 1991, patients freedom of choice of doctors and the Adel Reform of 1992 which changed financial responsibility for elderly care from the county councils to the municipalities (Bergman, 1998). For the purpose of this chapter, however, the Stockholm Model and the Family Doctors Legislation (Prop 1994/95) are selected for closer examination.

THE STOCKHOLM MODEL

In January 1992, the Stockholm County Council responsible for approximately 1.7 million people embarked on a new way of financing and organizing health care. The Stockholm Model was introduced to strengthen the position of patients in their choice of care, and to provide more effective health care (Hakansson, 1994; Quaye, 2001). Within this model, an internal market system was created separating hospitals from the county councils as purchasers and producers of health care. Hospitals and doctors were paid for medical activities in accordance with a new reimbursement system. Prices were determined through an elaborate points system based on diagnostic-related groups (DRGs) that result in a standard maximum price list (Glennerster and Matsaganis, 1994). Several aspects of the Stockholm Reform were included in the 1994 national Family Doctor's Legislation which had the goal of encouraging privatization of primary care physicians. Section 5 of the Act allowed each family doctor to keep a list of patients served and remuneration paid to family doctors consisted of a fixed amount per patient (capitation) (Quaye, 1997).The goal was to reduce the use of hospital resources by strengthening the primary care sector since 80 percent of Swedes were going directly to hospitals for medical care (Hakansson,1999). However this legislation has since been repealed by the Social Democrats.

In a review of the Stockholm Model, Bergman reported that the essential features of both privatization of primary health care and its reimbursement have been retained in systems run by each county council. The Swedish government and the Federation of County Councils also introduced the "care guarantee" for some medical operations (Bergman,1998). The goals were to ensure that patients received treatment within three months of diagnosis. Barring that, counties were to be held financially liable.

The Adel Reform of 1992 also transferred responsibility for the care of the elderly from the county council to the municipalities. The municipalities under this reform were given the responsibility for establishing special residential forms of service and care for those who needed it. It is also the duty of the municipalities to provide help and medical services for the elderly in their special housing. In addition, the municipalities incur the financial costs of acute medical and other geriatric care (Federation of County Councils, 1993).

Evaluators of these reforms have concluded that productivity has increased and efficiency has improved (Jonsson,1996;Quaye,1997;Bergman,1998; Whitehead and Varde,1997 and Hakansson,1999). Hakansson in his discussion of productivity after the introduction of the Stockholm Model and the DRG-based reimbursement payment system concluded that Swedish inpatient care increased by 8 percent, day surgery by 50 percent and outpatient visits by 15 percent (Hakansson,1999). Similarly, Bruce and Jonsson's eval-

Table 4.1. Percentage Change in Output, Costs and Productivity in Somatic Acute Care for Five Counties Utilizing Per Case Payment Versus Group of 14 Counties with Traditional Annual Budgets (Control) 1990–1993

Control Group	Model Counties				
	Sormland	Stockholm	Darlana	Bohuslan	Orebro
Output	+9.2	+11.0	-0.8	+7.2	+7.7
Costs -3.4	-4.3	-4.0	-11.4	-8.7	+7.0
Productivity +2.4	+14.1	+16.0	+12.1	+17.4	+0.7

Source: Bruce & Jonsson 1996, Hakansson 1999

Table 4.2. Output and Annual Percentage Change in Productivity for Somatic Acute Care Hospitals Stockholm County 1992–1996

Year	Output	DRG/KOKs	Productivity	Productivity/DRG/KOKs
1992	+7.0	N/A	+8.0	N/A
1993	0.0	N/A	+11.0	N/A
1994	+3.0	N/A	-8.0	N/A
1995	-7.0	-4.0	-3.0	-4.0
1996	-4.0	-2.0	-8.0	-1.0

DRG: diagnostic-related group
KOKS: classification in outpatient surgical care
Source: Hakansson, 1999; Charpentier and Samuelson, 1999

uation of productivity between five so-called model counties and 14 control counties concluded that the model counties increased their productivity more than the control counties. The productivity was 14.1 percent, 16 percent, 12.1 percent, 17.4 percent and 7 percent for the five model counties (Hakansson, 1999). Table 4.1 summarizes this trend.

In his paper, Hakansson, quoting the Charpentier and Samuelson study of 1999, reported that "Total output measured as the number of discharges in inpatient care and the number of physician visits in ambulatory care during 1992–96 increased during 1994–96." Table 4.2 summarizes this trend.

In their 1994 study, Svensson and Garelius reported that there was no evidence that the Stockholm Model had led to cream-skimming of patients, DRG creep, or over treatment of patients (Svensson and Garelius,1994).

RESEARCH METHODS AND DATA COLLECTION

To explore current views of Stockholm physicians, politicians, and health economists on these internal market reforms seven years after their introduction, a study was conducted in Stockholm in 1999. Of particular interest were in the views of physicians, especially, primary physicians and heads of hospital departments. This study obtained:

- views on the repeal of the national legislation on family doctor's practice by the Social Democratic government and its continuing in some counties; and the effect of the primary care physicians on medical costs;
- relationship between specialists and primary care physicians;
- current work settings and their degree of professional autonomy experienced by physicians before and after the introduction of the Stockholm Model and
- views of physicians, health economists, and politicians on the development of DRG-reimbursement for inpatient care and

- the impact, if any, of the cost-control mechanisms on the practice of medicine;
- career and job satisfaction among physicians;
- future trends and needs in Swedish health care (See Appendix for Interview Schedule).

The data were obtained in the summer of 1999 from in-depth interviews with fifteen(15) primary care physicians, four (4) heads of hospital departments (surgery) five(5) Stockholm County Council members and four (4) national health economists (N=28). Because the goal was to explore diverse perspectives, I deliberately utilized the snowball sampling strategy to reach particular health care provider populations. The interviews were conducted at clinics and hospitals, Stockholm County Council offices, and at the National Board of Health and Welfare. Each interview was conducted in English and audio taped with permission and transcribed. The interviews lasted between one and two hours. A content analysis was performed to uncover major themes on the interview transcripts.

VIEWS ON DRGS SEVEN YEARS AFTER THEIR INTRODUCTION

We found respondents well aware that financial incentives introduced through performance-based (DRGs) reimbursement exist in Stockholm. The Stockholm Model, which most of our respondents cited specifically, is still more or less in practice. Hospitals are still paid according to DRG in inpatient care. The cornerstone of the reform, according to key politicians from the Stockholm County Council was to "ensure efficiency, productivity, accessibility, and choice for patient." Stockholm is reported to rely heavily on the use of DRGs with about 70 percent of all acute care funds (total budget of 9 billion Swedish crowns) allocated based on the DRGs. The four hospital heads of departments reported that they were reimbursed by the County Council through 100 percent DRG.

The department heads also confirmed that productivity and efficiency have increased in their hospitals. As one head of department declared, "Under the old system, having more patients waiting for surgery was the best thing, but now, less waiting length is the best." Another head of department stated:

> When I started here [in this hospital] we had a waiting list of almost one thousand patients. My understanding was that for hospitals to get more money, they had to show that they had patients waiting for a long time. I think most of the clinics still work that way but I decided that to be efficient means we reduce the number on the waiting lists. My predecessor said that [cutting down] the wait-

ing lists is like taking all the safety nets away, but I thought that is the only way to survive. In the long run it has been confirmed because the politicians and the general practitioners feel this is good.

When respondents were asked whether they thought using DRG is a good system for allocating health resources, overwhelmingly politicians, physicians and health economists considered it the best system available so far. This view is consistent with earlier studies. Forsberg reported that 60 percent of her sampled physicians felt the DRG was a good system (personal interview, August 1999). One head of department reported that," The DRG system is the best system we have now. This is better than the global budget system."

While most of the respondents generally were in favor of the DRG system, several voiced concerns. For instance, a surgeon, in answer to the question as to whether the DRG system is a good system for allocating health care resources, had this to say:

Well, I think they are still struggling with the DRGs. I am not so tuned in to the details of the system, but there are always some winners and losers in that kind of system. There have been a lot of protests from large hospitals that they are not being reimbursed adequately, and that is damaging to their research. But I have not heard of any alternative system. I think one of the questions is how to pay for the services provided through telemedicine [diagnosis and advice over the telephone].

A general physician, who until three years before the interview was a surgeon in one of the hospitals, reported his experience with DRGs. " I worked with the DRG system at another hospital from 1993 to 1995. It involved a lot of paperwork for every single doctor. I think it is most important that the patient treatment is not influenced by money. I do think it is the right system for allocating health care resources."

As one of the health economist, "The DRG system is regulated only by the contracts made between purchasers and providers and as a result the "economic incentives are destroyed by the regulatory system so there is no incentive to work hard. This is one of the reasons why physicians do not like it very much."

A few of the respondents claimed that physicians' attitudes are changing and that they are more cost-conscious than before. One general physician stated, in response to a question about his experiences with DRGs that:

I think [DRGs] are fairly good. The problem has been that [even with DRGs] hospitals have not managed to keep within their budgets and they have been subsidized by the county council. Since we became a corporation, we have operated within our budget and yet we are not allowed to expand. We think we are the only hospital operating with profit and we should be allowed to do more to increase our productivity, but the county council is not prepared to do so.

EFFECTS OF PRIVATIZATION OF FAMILY MEDICINE

Under the Family Doctor's Act of 1994 family physicians were allowed to establish their own private practices and were paid on a fee-for-service basis without negotiating contracts with the County Council. In my research on the effects of this reform on physicians' practice, general practitioners reported an enhanced social and economic status within the medical profession (Quaye, 1997). As already mentioned, this legislation was abolished by the incoming Social Democratic government in 1995.

It has been argued that although the emergence of the primary care physician as a separate specialty is a significant innovation in the medical division of labor, it is not clear that the primary care physician has made a decisive contribution to improving health care in Sweden. In any case, under the Family Doctors legislation, the family physician seemed sure that they were seeking increased responsibility, respect, and autonomy in the medical decision process. A re-examination of family physicians and their views on the repealed legislation does provide valuable information for understanding the current role of primary physicians in overall health care delivery in Sweden.

Primary care physicians were asked about their views on privatizing the primary health care sector. Most of the primary care physicians have positive impressions of the privatization process. Primary care physicians who currently are in private practice praised the legislation. As one of them reported "We were lucky we did it when they [conservatives] were in power." Some specifically mentioned that the reform enhanced their social and economic status.

Some complained that the new legislation created more work for them and when asked whether the system is still in force even under the current Social Democratic administration, most felt some versions do exist in counties with Conservative Party majorities. While there is no formal legislation, in several parts of Stockholm there is a campaign to encourage general practitioners to go private. In fact, this applies to anyone within the county council's purview who works in primary care, psychiatry, and nursing care. The National Board of Health and Welfare would like to see some controlled trials of this policy which was also endorsed by the politicians interviewed.

RELATIONSHIP BETWEEN SPECIALISTS AND PRIMARY CARE PHYSICIANS

The majority of physicians interviewed reported good professional relationships with their colleagues. But primary care physicians were more likely to report that this relationship could be better. Most of them reflected on their status vis-a vis the medical division of labor in Sweden. One primary care physician noted that, " I think it is good but it could be better. They think we are second-class citizens or something. If you know and work with them, it is okay. But there is still a general feeling that they see themselves as better than we are." Another primary care physician stated that, "They send the problematic patients to us. There is collegiality when it comes to working with patients, except that they tend to dump difficult patients on us." One primary care physician remarked that, "It has been very good all the years. Those of us who work in this clinic are highly respected because we have such difficult cases."

The head of a department in one hospital asserted that the nature and degree of collegiality differs from one Stockholm district to another. In northeastern Stockholm, for example, hospital doctors have better working relationships with primary care physicians. He stated, "We have good relations. We depend on their referrals, and we work very hard to maintain good relations with them. We do have regular meetings with representatives of primary care physicians to discuss the services we provide and how best we can improve what we currently offer."

What is clear from respondents' comments was the need for better coordination in the delivery of health services. As one primary care physician put it, "We are gatekeepers, and because the system is not working at the level it should be, we should have better relationships between primary care physicians and specialists in hospitals."

WORKING CONDITIONS

On average, primary care physicians reported seeing between 15 and 20 patients every working day. They also make some house calls, which means about 350 patients every month.

Most reported that they are generally satisfied with their work. A family physician in private practice stated that, "In general, I am satisfied with my work. I do not feel stressed out. I have few patients with severe problems and I am also satisfied with my personal income. Our incomes are higher than government-employed [county council] primary care physicians."

When heads of departments were asked to evaluate the working conditions for their colleagues, they reported that they believe there is a small change for the better. They argued that hospital doctors have higher salaries or at least have the potential to earn more than they used to. One mentioned that they do use a bonus system linked to hospital performance.

But some of the respondents expressed their dissatisfaction with the health care delivery system. They reported that salaries are low. A surgeon noted that, "The Stockholm area has always been well-supplied with doctors, and this has made the average salary in Stockholm lower than in other parts of Sweden. This is likely to change, given the shortage of surgeons. Two primary care physicians gave especially negative views of their work. One of them reported that the "working conditions are poor and they see too many patients."

Yet, when physicians were asked if they would recommend the profession to other members of their family, most said that they have no reservation in doing so. Most felt generally satisfied with what they do. A primary care physician stated that, "It is interesting work. I have great fun all the time, although it is very difficult at times. I would prefer to have time off to do research. But another respondent replied, "I ask myself that question. I am not quite sure, because I do not like it. If I have a daughter, I am not sure I will recommend that. Before I became a physician, I went to business school. If you are a businesswoman, you have more freedom."

When physicians were asked to discuss how best the Swedish health care system could reduce costs, there was unanimous agreement that the role of primary physicians should be expanded. In particular, all primary care physicians not surprisingly believed that they should have a well-defined role as gatekeepers. One commented that to meet people's health needs, "' Fundamental changes must occur in the health care system and the family doctor must play a central role." Another respondent stated," I think there are several solutions, but I am a primary care physician and if you look globally you have to focus on primary health care to reduce costs in the hospitals. But the politicians have not had the will to do so." Another physician mentioned that "Being the primary-care first line of contact in taking care of patients, we have constant contact with the patients. Our role is to sort out their conditions."

One primary care physician in private practice stated, "I think primary health care should be private. Primary care doctors can provide the best care for their patients and they can decide what they want to do." A surgeon mentioned that, "The family doctors, psychiatrists, and pathologists in Sweden have very low status compared with other specialties. For this reason, the government should enhance the status of primary care physicians."

Respondents mentioned the need to make their work more attractive through salary increases but also reduced workload per doctor, more respect from their peers, and better specification of professional roles. But on a negative note, a primary care physician noted that:

> I am really pessimistic. I wonder if the government really wants more GPs or not. They do not seem to encourage our practice, even though they say they do.

I do not think they do. I do not know if our status has grown any. In some respects, I guess it has, but I do not know. The work I am doing is very important. It is very important for the personal life of our patients.

FUTURE TRENDS AND NEEDS

Several respondents felt that current internal market systems will continue and that we are more likely to see decreasing roles for the national government and greater decentralization of the health care system. Some also expressed the feeling that there will be more privatization and sales of county hospitals such as St. Goran's hospital in Stockholm. The respondents concluded that while the use of the DRG system is not perfect, it is by far the most efficient way found so far for allocating health care resources. I will explore this further in the next chapter with a follow-up study. Respondents drew attention to the need for collaboration between counties, especially in southern Sweden, in the delivery of health care. As one politician pointed out, " We should find ways to streamline our hospitals. One proposal would be to have smaller hospitals closer to people and have about eight or nine big hospitals spread throughout Sweden." When asked to reflect on future needs and trends in health care a head of department suggested that, " I think we will have problems with the elderly and we do not have enough doctors. Most of the doctors will leave but they will come back and I think the status of the medical profession will be very good."

From the perspective of health economists, two concluded that the system is more likely to be privatized because the county councils are not capable of dealing with these challenges. As one health economist noted, " I think that what remains to be seen is how we are preparing for this huge shortage of doctors. There is another question, of whether we should bring more doctors from outside Sweden or try to promote preventive health."

Another health economist said, " I do think that the system is changing in a way that we will see greater responsibility for all doctors, and there will be connections between what we produce and how we are paid. I think incentives are good for ensuring efficiency and productivity and that the health care system will work better." One of the surgeons interviewed commented that " For the moment, the system is cost-effective and definitely people are getting the care they need. The problem is that we are seeing escalating cost. The real problem, though, is that doctors and nurses are poorly paid compared with their contemporaries in Europe." A primary care physician reflected on the fact that money is distributed in the wrong way. When asked to explain this further, she declared," I cannot understand why teenagers have free access to health care. They are usually healthy, and yet there are a lot of people who are ill and unhealthy who cannot go to the hospital because it costs too much." A clinic chief argued that, " we have to be more concerned about our work and to be more cost-conscious but still take care of all our patients."

CONCLUSION

By examining the perspectives of physicians, politicians, and health economists on recent changes in the Swedish health care system, the research focused on health care reforms in Stockholm, but it nevertheless represents part of internal market reforms important to understanding an analysis of the various regional changes in the Swedish health care systems. The findings suggest that most physicians are generally satisfied with their working conditions and look favorably on the use of the DRG-based reimbursement system as an effective way to allocate health care resources. Most of the respondents were supportive of the various market reforms strategies, including the privatization of St. Goran's Hospital in Stockholm. As one remarked, " If what is good for St. Goran is good for Stockholm, then we should see more hospitals taking that route."

This investigation also underscores the significant role that politics play in the Swedish health delivery system. As mentioned earlier, most of the privatization initiatives—The Stockholm Model, care guarantees and the use of DRGs—were initiated under the national Conservative administration and portions of it have been maintained by the Social Democratic Party government. The current wave of privatizations in counties that has Conservative majorities has raised the important connection between what goes on at the local and the national level.

The most intriguing aspect of the Swedish experience is its degree of decentralization. Counties can and will continue to experiment with several different health care modalities. Ultimately, the country as a whole will gain from such experimentation if the experiments are properly evaluated and refined to deal with economic changes as they occur.

What is clear, though, is that in all this, the role of the primary care physician in the medical division of labor is uncertain. Yet, although it has been argued that the emergence of the primary care physician is a significant innovation in the medical division of labor, it is not clear that primary care physicians have made a unique contribution to health care in Sweden. Indeed, there have been relatively few studies done on the potential role of primary care physicians in the changing overall health care system in Sweden.

This chapter has essayed a contribution to the comparative study of health and health care in developed countries. The investment of the Swedish government and counties in developing the role of primary care physicians as gatekeepers is laudable and long overdue. The primary care physician's role, due to its potential benefit as an agent of cost control, is clearly important. Yet, as we better understand the changes taking place, an understanding of the perspectives of physicians, politicians, and health economists will become increasingly useful. The next chapter focuses on DRGs as a special issue in health care financing, and will explore the extensive discussion of the role of this reimbursement system in the delivery of care, and assess to what extent this payment system is undermining the Swedish goal of equal access to health for all as mandated by the Swedish Medical Health Care Act.

Chapter Five

Diagnostic Related Groups (DRGs): Special Case of Reform in Sweden

Much has been written about the role of diagnostic-related groups as a cost-effective measure in health care. In the United States, this system goes back to April 1983 when the U.S. legislature, in an attempt to control mounting Medicare costs, created the Medicare Prospective Payment System (PPS). Prior to this time, Medicare gave hospitals a cost-based blank check honoring whatever bills hospitals submitted for payment. In a nutshell, the Medicare payment system had been based on a retrospective payment system. Such a system had the perverse incentive of encouraging hospitals to increase their overheads which ultimately led to higher costs for Medicare (Fetter, 1991).

According to Richard Averill and Michael Kalison (1989), as a result of the PPS Medicare payments, the total cost to hospitals of their services increased by 19 percent. Hospitals had had no incentive to hold down costs or maximize efficiency. They reported that, "The Medicare hospital deductible [had] increased at a rate far higher than beneficiaries [could] afford or [were] willing to pay and it was estimated that if the current spending continued, the rapid rate of increase in hospital costs would endanger the solvency of the Medicare Trust Fund." (p.207). Thus the establishment of the DRG-based Medicare Prospective Payment System, according to Bardsley, Coles, and Jenkins (1989), was motivated by provisions in the earlier Tax Equity and Fiscal Responsibility Act of 1982 (TEFRA) (PL 97-248). This law was designed to cap the amount of Medicare money available for hospital-based care "(p.38).

The benefits of this payment system, according to Averill and Kalison (1989), are that:

1. The payment rates are established in advance and are fixed for the fiscal period to which they apply.

2. The payment rates are not automatically determined by the hospital's past or current actual cost.
3. The prospective payment rates are payment in full.
4. The hospitals retain the profit or suffer a loss resulting from the difference between the payment rate and the hospitals costs (p.208).

The goal of this system is to have hospitals respond to the financial incentives engineered by this payment system by producing cost-effective service without reducing the quality of care.

In practice, though, since physicians' behavior contributes to higher hospital costs as, the physicians are critical to any cost-control strategy. After all, in situations where a payment to a hospital exceed its costs, there will be greater pressure on their part to manipulate the system. The so called, "DRG-creep"—which is the arbitrary changing of the assignment of codes for payment in order to optimize DRG-payment assignments of cost. In this way, the underlying cost-assignment structure allows any additional diagnosis or procedure to elevate the patient into a new and more expensive category.

This is particularly serious concern because of "outliers." Outlier is a patient who can be assigned to a DRG but has an extremely high or an extremely low cost or length of stay relative to most patients in the same DRG (Averill and Kalison, 1989:214). It is estimated that about 2 percent of U.S. Medicare patients are considered outliers. As the authors point out with respect to "high" outliers, "such atypical patients can be very expensive to treat and must be recognized as exceptions in the calculation of the DRG payment amounts. Failure to do so for high-cost outliers would have severe consequences for a hospital's financial viability."

Specifically, DRGs are defined as "a patient classification scheme which provides a means of relating the types of patients a hospital treats to the costs incurred by the hospital by classifying patients based on diagnosis. It is a system for describing the types of patients discharged from acute care hospitals" (Fetter, 1991: 5).

INTERNATIONAL COMPARISONS OF DRGS

In countries where DRGs have been introduced, the effect has been immediate. Among its benefits, DRGs provide a better description of the desired end product of a hospital's activities—and therefore provide a much better indication of how money is being spent in providing care (Averill and Kalison, 1989:164). It can also provide routine and immediate comparative assessment of the financial implications of treating different types of patients, and make possible international comparisons as well. Beyond that, DRGs have resulted in reduction in the length of stays in hospitals and also led to reduced admissions to hospitals.

In assessing the future of DRGs, Coles and Jenkins (1989:56), quoted Iglehart: "Looked at another way, hospitals also will have a new incentive to under-serve patients, the same incentive that health maintenance organizations have by virtue of their fixed, prospective form of payment."

They point out that "the current system includes incentive for hospitals to operate on those patients who have (surgical DRGs) have higher costs assigned to them at the expense of less-profitable patients), thus resulting in uneven provision of services" (p.170).

WHAT HAS BEEN THE SWEDISH EXPERIENCE WITH DRGS?

Discussion in the use of DRGs in Swedish health care system started in 1984 with the publication of two articles and an editorial in the Swedish Medical Association journal. This was followed the following year by a conference on DRGs organized by the Swedish Planning and Rationalizing Institute (SPRI) in collaboration with the Health Systems Management Group at Yale University (Hakansson and Gavelin, 1999). The result of that effort led to the first DRG databases from the Stockholm County Council and the municipality of Gothenburg. These databases consisted of information on 512,000 discharges from 22 hospitals. The initial goal was to assess the feasibility of using DRGs from hospital data to evaluate if this model could be successfully used to gauge length of stay by different types of patients in hospitals. In clinical studies led by Dr. Carl-Axel Nilsson in 1988, the Swedish DRGs were used on obstetrics and gynecological patients. Between 1989 and 1994, this model was extended to cover: general surgery and urology, internal medicine, and infectious diseases (Hakansson and Gavelin, 1999). In a randomized study by SPRI of 432 Ob-gyn discharges from 31 hospitals, 21 percent of the discharges had errors in diagnosis or procedure code. And 9 percent of these discharges led to a wrong DRG assignment. In a follow-up study of 482 discharges in general surgery and urology, 18 percent of all inliers and 34 percent of all outliers were assigned to a wrong DRG. In another study carried out in hospitals in southern Stockholm in 1994, the data suggested that 25.4 percent of the discharges had erroneously registered diagnoses and procedure codes (Hakansson and Gavelin, 1999).

In a follow up study conducted by the National Board of Health and Welfare of the Center of Patient Classification System, Serden and Lindqvist reported that as a result of the introduction of the DRG system, hospital with such prospective payment systems had a higher number of secondary diagnoses per case than before the introduction of DRG-based management systems, suggesting that the introduction of DRG have had a perverse incentive to increase the number of secondary diagnoses. While the authors attribute this increase to the change in the coding system from ICD-9 to ICD-10 in 1997, they were actually not able to ascertain whether this factor contributed to the large number of secondary diagnoses. As they reported, there was no question that the implementation of a DRG-based payment system gave strong incentives for increasing the number of diagnoses per patient (Serden and Lindqvist, 2001).

In a comprehensive study conducted by Forsberg, Axelsson, and Arnetz (2000) on the effects of performance-based reimbursement in Swedish health care, the authors "examined whether performance-based reimbursement had affected physicians' attitudes and behavior towards improved effectiveness or not" (p.3). They compared the perspectives of physicians employed by the Stockholm County Council, where the DRG reimbursement system had been introduced, and 11 other county councils in various regions of Sweden without the performance-based system. They reported that a majority of Stockholm physicians were supportive of this payment system (57%), and the majority of the sampled physicians believed that their own clinic had become more efficient in terms of shorter waiting time for medical examinations than before the introduction of the DRG system. The authors pointed out that one immediate effect of the DRG system was reduction in average length of hospital stay in all counties polled, although the reduction was more significant in Stockholm County than the other counties. More physicians in Stockholm than in the 11 other counties reported that the number of premature discharges from hospitals had increased (72% in Stockholm, compared with 60% in the 11 other counties), and that 24 percent of physicians in Stockholm compared with 11 percent of physicians in the other 11 counties reported, that patients were often discharged prematurely from the hospital or clinic. While the researchers concluded that the data did not "support the belief that the quality of care has deteriorated, they found that the quality of care in certain districts of Stockholm had deteriorated (p.108).

In a follow-up study in 2001, I interviewed physicians in Stockholm on the impact of the DRG reimbursement payment system on aspects of their work. What follows is the result of that study, compared to my findings in 1999.

SWEDISH PHYSICIANS' ATTITUDES: A FOLLOW-UP STUDY ON DRGS

In the past decade, rising health care expenditures have forced many countries to institute new ways of financing health care. In nearly all countries in Europe, national governments initiated policies geared towards providing health care efficiently through the introduction of market-oriented reforms (Quaye, 2001).

In Sweden, approximately half of the 26 county councils have instituted a system of independent purchasers and providers, and introduced a performance-based reimbursement system in the form of diagnostic-related groups (Saltman, 1995; Forsberg, 2001).

This section examines more specifically the impact of financial incentives on Swedish health care and explores how physicians' behavior is affected by cost-control measures. What is of particular interest is to look at Sweden as a welfare state in which health care is the responsibility of the public sector (Hakansson,1994). Examining what appears to be a much more liberal system that than that of the United States provides a good contrast for international comparative analyses. Given the Swedish differences from the United States in health care ideologies, that is the Swedish principles of solidarity, equity, and public control as contrasted with the private free-market health care financing typical of the United States, one would expect to see a different response to economic incentives among Swedish physicians than among physicians in the United States. But are they really different?

In 1992, Stockholm County introduced a performance-based reimbursement system where 100 percent of the hospital budget (except teaching and research) is based on hospital outcomes for patients (Forsberg, 2001). As Forsberg (2001:8) reported, "the case-based financing system and performance is measured by hospital discharge based on the DRG point system." These reforms entailed three principles: the purchaser/provider split, money payment to providers budgeted for care based on the characteristics of the population in the served area, and the introduction of an internal market system for health services. These reforms have brought into question the effects of economic incentives on physicians' attitudes and behavioral choices in the exercise of their professional clinical decision making, and raised the question of whether this approach has undermined the professional integrity of Swedish physicians.

PURPOSE OF STUDY

The specific issues raised by this study are:

- the extent to which the internal market reforms have over time affected the views and behaviors of physicians as they reflect on their working conditions;

- health care providers' experiences with the use of diagnostic-related groups (DRGs) as a payment system for hospitals; and
- career aspirations and job satisfaction as influenced by the effect of DRGs.

In exploring physicians' behavior in response to the new payment methodologies, I reviewed the pattern of these recent changes internationally in reimbursement strategies.

We considered how these structural changes might intersect with the specific designs of the Swedish health care system.

Studies have shown that such financial incentives do influence medical decision making (Hillman et al.,1989; Forsberg, 2001).

As clearly demonstrated in the literature, physicians' services are the second largest item in personal health care expenditure, accounting for 19.5 percent (or $761 per capita) of health care expenditure in the United States., 16.4 percent in Germany, and 12.2 percent in Sweden (Anderson and Poullier, 1999).

The DRG system introduced into health systems internationally was designed to provide physicians and hospitals with incentives to improve the efficiency and cost-effectiveness of health care services. Because savings derived from caring for patients at a cost less than the DRG payment become profits for hospitals, providers are encouraged to avoid over-treatment of patients and to limit the unnecessary medical procedures associated with the traditional fee-for-service systems (Davis et al.,1990; Franks et al., 1992). It is equally true that caring for patients at a cost greater than the DRG payment rate translates into a loss for hospitals. In response, this induces hospitals to "skimp" on the possible services they offer leading to what Taira and Taira (1991) refer to as "patient dumping" and Steinberg (1997) as "silent rationing." There is also a strong incentive to discharge patients as early as possible, with some patients likely to be discharged prematurely, leading to poor outcomes or increased hospital readmission rates (Davis et al.,1990).

In the Stockholm model, the DRG system was first introduced in five specialties: surgery, urology, orthopedics, obstetrics and gynecology (Hakansoon,1994).

In this study, we asked questions based on the analysis of possible consequences of such reforms for physicians. For instance, since a majority of physicians in Sweden receive none of the capped reimbursement for procedures, and are salaried, we expected to see some patterns of physicians' under-use of services for patients because of financial considerations, and constraints on hospital reimbursement. After all, "The gate-keeping role has come to simply mean the medically limited and bureaucratic function of opening or closing the gate on high cost medical services." (Frank, Nutting, and Clancy, 1991:424).

42   *Chapter Five*

METHOD AND DATA COLLECTION

These research data come from a survey mailed to physicians randomly selected from three major hospitals in Stockholm. Subjects were asked about their specialty, years of practice, medical practice conditions as well as the impact of cost-control measures on their clinical decision making. We asked questions about their arrangements with their hospital and whether these included some form of financial incentive in the form of a bonus. They were also asked on a Likert scale from 1= "strongly agree" to 5= "strongly disagree" whether they felt pressure from heads of medical departments and hospital administrators to limit patient services and whether they felt such pressures compromised patients' care. Other questions focused on physicians' career aspirations and their communicating these to their immediate relatives.

Physicians were asked to rate their own overall knowledge of the Stockholm Model, and to evaluate whether the effects of the Stockholm Model had been discussed in their medical departments. They were also asked to rate their current practice situation and to assess whether the hospital's economic performance had affected their work situation.

The questionnaires were distributed between May and August of 2001 to 100 randomly selected physicians in active practice in Stockholm County. The response rate was 46 percent.

DATA ANALYSIS

The questionnaire was developed from a systematic review of the literature on financial incentives in health care and from previous interviews with Stockholm physicians in 1999.

The questionnaire was constructed first in English and then translated into Swedish. The questionnaire was tested on a pilot group of three physicians and two health economists. The data were analyzed using an SPSS statistical package. (To investigate bivariate relationship among variables, we used cross-tabulations and chi-square tests of significance. The small sample size made further analysis impossible).

RESULTS

We received responses from 46 of the 100 physicians contacted. Of these respondents, 48 percent were heads of departments and or deputy hospital clinic

Table 5.1. Demographics and Practice Information Physicians' Respondents (Stockholm, 2001)

Gender	Percentage(%)
Male	81.0
Female	19.0
Total	100.0
Years of Pracice	*Percentage (%)*
0–10	32.6
11–21	37.0
22–31	23.9
401	4.3
N/A	2.2
Total	100.0
Medical Specialty	*Percentage (%)*
Hospital Clinic/Deput Chief	47.9
Internal Medicine	12.5
Surgery	22.9
Others	16.7
Total	100.0
Age	*Percentage (%)*
30–39	12.8
40–49	48.9
50–59	31.9
60–69	6.4
Total	100.0

chiefs, 13 percent were general internists, and 23 percent were surgical specialists. A total of 33 percent reported having worked for the Stockholm County less than ten years. Almost two-thirds had worked as physicians for 11 years or more (see Table 5.1).

FINANCIAL INCENTIVES IN HEALTH CARE AND EFFECTS ON HEALTH CARE

When respondents were asked about how much they know about the Stockholm Model and whether the effects of the model have been discussed in their respective hospital or clinic, 34 percent of the respondents answered yes. Twenty-seven percent reported that prioritization of different patients' care had changed. Thirty-nine percent reported that they often discussed profitable patients in their clinic. This suggests that the effect of cost control strategies through the DRG system have affected the way these Swedish physicians practice medicine. Respondents reported an increase in productivity and efficiency as a result of the system.

This finding is consistent with a study by Forsberg (2001:30) who reported that, "Almost all [her] respondents surveyed considered their own clinic to have become efficient, not only through the incentive to increase the number of patients, but also by changing routines."

About 77 percent of the respondents declared that DRG payments are a good principle for health care and 42 percent saw DRGs as a good payment system for allocating health care resources in Sweden. See Table 5.2.

Table 5.2. Physicians' Views on DRG Payment System, Stockholm, 2001

Response	Percentage (%)
Yes	34.0
No	31.9
Don't know	23.4
Total	100.0

Has prioritization of cases changed at your hospital/clinic?

Yes	26.9
No	46.2
Don't know	26.9
Total	100.0

Is DRG payment a good prinicple for adequate health care?

Yes, very	57.7
Yes	19.2
Not very	11.6
Not at a ll	11.5
Total	100.0

Is DRG payment a good system for allocating medical care?

Yes, very good	38.5
Yes, good	3.8
Not very good	34.6
Not at all good	15.4
N/A	7.7
Total	100.0

WORK SITUATION AND AUTONOMY

When physicians were asked if they felt the economic performance of the clinic affected their work situations, about fifty-eight percent reported it did. Somewhat less than half (42%) did not believe so. On the question of whether the financial incentive had an impact on their selection of patients, an overwhelming 92 percent responded that they did not make recommendations on that basis, suggesting that the effect has not led to any decrease in the quality of care provided. Indeed, when physicians were asked if they felt pressure to see more patients, 54 percent of our sample reported they did and 23 percent reported that such pressures to see more patients compromised patients' care. On the question of physicians' loss of professional autonomy, the majority of the respondents (70%) reported that physicians are losing control. About fifty-eight percent of the surveyed physicians reported that they were generally satisfied with their profession.

I also observed differences among physicians on the subject of whether they would recommend their profession to their immediate family members.

SATISFACTION

Half of the respondents reported that they were less than likely to recommend the profession to their immediate family members. Furthermore, younger physicians (30–39 years of age) were less satisfied with their work than those older physicians with less than ten years of practice (18%), compared to those with more years of practice.

Paradoxical way, I found that older physicians especially three (40–49 years of age) reported that they were less likely to recommend the medical profession to their relatives (40%), than younger physicians (30–39 years in age). Study found that internists were less satisfied with their work than surgeons or hospital clinic chiefs.

But surgical specialists were less likely to recommend the medical profession to their relatives than were internists. Specifically, about sixty-four percent of surgical specialists reported that they would not do so. This is illustrative, suggesting that the DRG system, in whatever form, is having a negative effect on the practice of medicine, since surgical specialists are those who work directly with the DRG system in hospitals and are therefore likely to be more influenced by these financial incentives. (See Table 5.3).

Table 5.3. Physicians' Autonomy and Satisfaction

Autonomy and satisfaction	Percentage (%)
Has prioritization of cases changed at your hospital/clinic?	
Yes, very much	38.5
Yes, much	19.2
Not much	27.9
Not at all	15.4
Total	100.0
Physicians' satisfaction with practice, Stockholm, 2001	
Great	8.7
Much	50.0
Not much	15.2
Not at all	6.5
N/A	19.6
Total	100.0

DISCUSSION

This chapter has reported on the perspectives of physicians in Stockholm County in 2001 and their experiences with the use of performance-based reimbursement in health care. The formulation of the questionnaire was guided by the following issues:

1. What is or should be the proper role of competitive behavior within a publicly financed health care system?
2. What are the consequences of the use of DRGs in Sweden for patient care and service delivery?

Because the current changes in the Swedish health-care system are still emerging, and given the relatively short experiences with performance-based reimbursement (PBR) in health care, studies differ as to the extent to which these changes describe prior theory as opposed to seeking to discover the empirical phenomena in need of theoretical explanation. The results of this study confirm Forsberg's (2001) extensive study on the effects of PBR on the quality of care. As Forsberg (2001:23) observed, " The PBR system did . . . strengthen the incentive to increase efficiency and did lead to the increase in the number of premature discharges from hospitals."

Her findings are generally consistent cross-nationally and not unique to Sweden in showing that the degree of satisfaction with PBR is related to such factors as age, years of practice, and physician type of specialty.

This study has several limitations. First, it is limited by the small sample. Second, since we did not ask our respondents directly about the impact of these measures on the delivery of care, it was difficult to determine whether their responses were a direct outcome of their own particular practice situations and not necessarily about the wider effects of the PBR system. Finally, a broader approach, comparing the experiences of physicians in other Swedish counties without the PBR system would have yielded better understanding of the role of financial incentives in health. Nevertheless, our findings generally support the claim that the PBR system in Sweden has, and will continue to have, an impact on doctoring in Sweden in the future.

Chapter Six

Is the Swedish Welfare State in Retreat?: Current Trends in Swedish Health Care

In the two decades, Sweden, like other European countries, has experimented with different health care financing modalities. In Stockholm County, for example, the use of a performance-based reimbursement system has been studied and extensively discussed by Swedish scientists and scholars. A careful review of these studies suggest that, on the whole, these market reforms have achieved their goals of efficiency and productivity in health services while simultaneously creating the kinds of incentives necessary for reducing inefficiencies by encouraging competition among health care providers.

My previous study reported in Chapter 4 explored the perspectives of Swedish physicians, politicians, and health economists seven years after the introduction of the so-called Stockholm Model.

> The majority of respondents reported that the financial incentives introduced through performance-based reimbursements do exist in Stockholm County and that productivity and efficiency had increased over the period of investigation. Primary care physicians voiced support for the privatization process in health care delivery. Most physicians reported that they were generally satisfied with their own work conditions. Over ninety percent of our respondents supported the use of diagnostic-related groups (Quaye, 2001).

Three years after the publication of that paper and 14 years since the introduction of market reforms, I wanted to explore the extent to which these changes have over time changed the nature of health care financing in Sweden, how these changes have affected the views of physicians in Sweden, and the impact of these reforms on the delivery and quality of care.

As in the previous study, we asked our respondents who are Stockholm health economists, private general practitioners, and hospital doctors the following questions:

- On their perspectives on the introduction of a performance-based reimbursement system, using diagnostic-related groups (DRGs) and an assessment of how well it has been practiced in their respective institutions;
- The extent to which internal market reforms have over time affected their working conditions and job satisfaction;
- The role of national policies on the health care delivery for the aged, and the consequences of the Adel Reform introduced in 1992;
- The current and future role of primary health care physicians in the overall health delivery system;
- Care guarantees and whether their introduction in November 2006 will affect the delivery of care by health care providers;

This paper reports the results of the study.

In recent years, economic incentives have become more and more important in health care, even in countries such as Sweden where health care is regarded as the responsibility of the welfare state (Forsberg, 2001). Approximately half of the 26 county councils in Sweden have instituted a system of health care purchasers and providers, and of performance-based reimbursement, measured according to the diagnostic-related groups (DRGs) system. In her study, Forsberg (2001) concluded that performance-based reimbursement has created clear incentives affecting physician decision-making resulting in an increase in attention to the quality of care. For a detailed discussion of the reforms starting in 1992, the reader should consult Quaye (2001).

METHODS

This study was designed to explore current views of Swedish physicians, Federation of County members, and health economists about these internal market reforms 13 years after their introduction. The data were obtained at work from in-depth interviews in English in the summer of 2005 with thirty-one Swedish health care personnel from Stockholm and Southern Sweden namely five health economists, eight heads of departments in hospitals or clinics, thirteen hospital specialists, plus four more general practitioners in private practice in Stockholm and two Federation of County Council members. They were selected using a snowball sampling technique in Stockholm County and Malmo and Lund University hospitals in Southern Sweden where DRGs are not used. Each interview was audiotaped in English with permission, and transcribed. The interview lasted between one and two hours. A content analysis on the transcripts was performed to determine major themes in the interviews.

RESULTS

Perspectives on Reimbursement in Health Care

Respondents were asked to discuss their experience with the use of financial incentives in health care, given the fact that the performance-based reimbursement system (DRG) has been used extensively in Stockholm and in the Skane region in Sweden. We wanted to assess the extent to which Swedish physicians have warmed up to this system of payment and whether its introduction has in any way undermined their medical performance expectations. We were particularly interested in exploring whether the financial incentives and the levels of productivity associated with the introduction of this reimbursement system was consistent with prevailing research on financial incentives in health care which shows that financial incentives do influence medical decision-making by physicians (Hillman et al., 1989).

Not surprisingly, all the health economists interviewed favored the use of the diagnostic related groups (DRGs) as an efficient mechanism for allocating health care resources. While they recognize the imperfections in the system (underutilization of services and DRG creep), they were unanimous in their evaluation that the introduction of the reimbursement system has worked well in Swedish health care by making the health care delivery system more efficient. They also mentioned that medical productivity had increased since the introduction of the DRG system. One of our health economist respondents stated that,

"Well, I think the [DRG] system is working well. The problem I see is that it has not been used widely in all hospitals across Sweden and the use of this system for outpatient care is not well developed."

In response to the question about why Sweden has been successful in decreasing health care cost, one health economist mentioned that the reduction in cost should be attributed in part to the effects of the DRG system. While he did not attribute the reduction only to the use of the DRG system, he was nevertheless emphatic in saying that the DRG system is a good system and should be further developed. He asserted that, "The DRG system is the best system so far in evaluating clinics, especially in hospitals, but of course there is a problem using it in primary care because it is tied to what you actually do and primary care does not lend itself to such measurements." To a question as to how widely the DRG system is used as a reimbursement system, another health economist pointed out that the system is not used in all Swedish counties, but only in Stockholm County, the Skane region, Vastra-Gotland region and Goteborg. He reported that the National Board of Health and Welfare is currently working on developing a national DRG weighting system to be used nationally. This, he felt, would allow for more accurate comparisons to be made across different counties.

By contrast, however, more than sixty-five percent of physicians interviewed did not support use of the DRG system. The strongest criticism of the DRG system came from primary care physicians in private practice and from hospital chiefs. In response to the question whether the DRG system is a good system for paying hospitals for what they do, a private general practitioner reported that, "No, I do not think it is a very good system because when I worked at the hospital in geriatrics many years ago, the hospital staff were looking at the patients and trying to find as many DRG points. Sometimes a patient coming from the hospital had been treated for urinary infection but did not have it."

When I followed up by asking if there were cases of wrong diagnoses, she responded yes. It is not always appropriate to treat an older patient for a urinary tract infection if she does not have any symptoms."

Another primary care practitioner in private practice claimed that the DRG system is not good because it is used wrongly. Asked to explain, she discussed DRG creep. "The hospital tries to get as many points as possible because the hospital is paid according to DRG points and such practices create problems." In theory, she states, "it is good, but in practice it is not working as it should."

As to whether the DRG system is good for allocating health care resources, a clinic chief in a major hospital in Stockholm declared that,

> No, I do not think so, because there are too many difficulties in how it is used. For example, at the intensive care unit, it is more expensive if you are forced to have acute or unplanned operations when patients come in and you are paid through the DRG system. Whereas if you are in private practice, you can choose patients that are less expensive or more healthy and hence better payment outcomes.

A specialist in urology reported that the DRG system is a complicated system set up for outpatients and there are many situations that treatments are not warranted and this leads to abuses in the system." Another hospital physician assessed the DRG system; "I think it has its advantages, although it generates a lot of administration, but it is one way to control cost. For me, the issue is the administration and the complicated way you have to put a tag on everything that you do and make sure you have the abbreviation for everything you do."

From the perspective of a urologist in private practice,

> The DRG system as used in Stockholm is not good. There are a lot of problems associated with its use. I remember, when they started the DRG system in Karolinska Hospital, in the beginning we did not receive the money we were promised because we did not register all the patients in DRG and then we paid a couple of nurses whose only job was to look over the medical diagnoses to get as much money as possible from each patient... So I think it is not a good system to be used in hospitals.

Another private general practitioner voiced concern that the DRG system is a system for cheating because "when the patients come from the hospital to my office, I see their papers and they do not have one diagnosis but twenty, and they always have this urinary tract infection because the more diagnoses the more they are paid, and I think this is ridiculous."

In an answer to the question about the effectiveness of using financial incentives in health care, including the DRG system, the chief of clinic at a major hospital responded by saying that,

> There are certainly a good deal of limitations in the system. It has been absolutely right to have the DRG system as a basis for describing production in the hospital. As you know, of course, there are more difficulties registering the output in the hospital and even the activities concerning the general practitioner. Certainly there are problems, but from the hospital point of view, the system is developing and it is very slow. But I do have difficulty seeing any other alternatives to the DRG system. Being a university hospital, we have specific problems concerning the DRG system because the case mix is highly specialized. That is partially taken care of, but not sufficiently so. Certainly, I think there is a drawback.

From the perspective of another hospital physician,

> The DRG system is reasonable, but I have been to hospitals in Dalarna and others in Sweden where the DRG system is not used and they take care of every patient that comes there. We have been living with the DRG system for such a long time that we feel it is okay and a reasonable system. We feel if we do a little more we could earn a little more.

The physicians' evaluation of the DRG system was well summed-up by one chief of clinic in a detailed response to the question as to the viability of the DRG system; he states that there will not be an answer to this question for another 50 years. He asserts,

> I am not sure, but I think the thing in the old days was we had a budget for each year, and that amount was sufficient no matter what we did. But when the DRG was introduced all of a sudden we were paid for what we did. So if we operated on more hernias or kidney stones, we got more money to cover the increased costs incurred for the increased work we did. And that was a positive thing because the waiting list dropped dramatically. But the DRG system as currently configured is not a good system for income-generating for hospitals, since each diagnostic-related group assessed contained several diagnoses and several different operations. So if a hospital specializes in some types of operations, those could be very generously paid by the DRG system. But if another hospital specializes in other diagnoses within the same DRG, then that hospital will have high costs and the income will not be enough to offset the cost.

To a follow-up question, on whether the DRG system would work if it were combined into one unit, he replied that:

> Well, since the case mix differs from hospital to hospital, it will still not work. If one hospital takes care of the most healthy patients with hernias as they get the same income as we do, who takes care of the more severely ill patients that demand more anesthesia or maybe even intensive care. The system is not precise enough to give an adequate income for each operation.

Elder Health Care Changes and Their Consequences (Adel Reform)

In 1992 the Adel Reform transferred the responsibility for the care of the elderly from the county councils to the municipalities. The municipalities under this reform were given the responsibility for establishing special residential forms of service and care for those who needed it. It is also the duty of the municipalities to operate help and medical services in this housing. As a result, the municipalities also incur the financial costs of acute medical and geriatric care (4).

We asked our respondents to assess the role of this reform on the health care delivery system. While about half of our respondents reported that the basic ideals of the reform were sound and have worked in some areas, even they raised concerns that the current system is not working to fully meet the need of the elderly population. One health economist, in answering whether the reform has worked, stated that, "Of course there are some who think that it has not been working and has created problems, since the doctors are not involved much in the nursing homes. But of course, this can easily be solved."

A similar sentiment was echoed by one head of clinic. She asserted that:

> The problem has always been policing the borders between the different health care systems. There are some good departments but at the borders of two systems

[county council and municipalities] there could be more effort made to coordinate their activities. For example, you have each department with its own budget and different demands so I think that can be a problem with coordination.

Another health economist respondent mentioned that,

The elderly care reform did have the effect that was wished for, since before the reform so many older and sick patients were lying in hospitals not in need of medical attention. The reforms made it easier for these patients to be transferred into the community, but maybe the care for these people is slightly not so good.

From the perspective of another health economist,

The Adel Reform was a good idea, but the benefits have not been as large as expected because the cooperation between the county council and the municipalities and the hospitals had not functioned well, so there has been a lot of tension between the municipalities and the hospitals. These are more financial problems than lack of staff in elderly care. The municipalities do not have the financial means and the competency to deal with the system. The municipalities are not allowed to have doctors employed but only nurses and paramedics. So to care for the elderly they have to depend on the county council doctors. So there is a lot of friction between the county councils and the municipalities, and also it is a field that does not attract too many doctors. It is not a problem now but it will be in the future.

Another health economist respondent mentioned that, of all the reforms introduced in the early 1990s, the Adel Reform is one that has not worked properly. When asked to elaborate, he stated that,

Now in some areas it is a no man's land since no one wants to take care of them. So I think when the reform was introduced they should have collapsed the role of the county councils with the municipalities, and because they did not do that, now they are fighting over who should take care of such matters. That is where the no-man's-land situation arises.

A private family care physician with over thirty-five years of medical practice, in response to a question about the elderly care reforms had this to say, "It has not worked as well as one would have hoped because the patients used to be in the nursing homes and now the county councils hires physicians to take care of them once a week. I think maybe the issue should be solved a little differently."

In a follow-up question about the impact of the reform on hospital discharge, and whether some patients have been sent home sooner than before, she responded by saying,

I think that is true, because it is always an economic question as to who is going to pay for the care, and I think more people need to be in a nursing home than at home. There are so many elderly who are being taken care of at home. And these are elderly who must be in a nursing home where they can get the help and the security that they need, but there are no rooms for them in the nursing home. I therefore think it is not working very well.

One Federation of County Councils official stated that:

I think it has worked, but no one is prepared to say that it has worked well with no problems. I think the tail end of it is that the elderly can get more services. But the political issue is how much one expects the elderly to request. There are more demands made on the municipalities but at the same time, the municipalities may not have the resources, so they cut down on the services they provide as well.

A clinic chief, in response to the question on impact of elderly care reform, declared even more firmly that:

No, the reform has not worked. It could certainly be improved. I think the question is how much this is related to this law. This has been, as I know, the problem because you have tension because the need for the hospitals to send patients back to the municipalities is great. Of course, the municipalities do not see the need as we do in the hospital and we have ongoing discussion with the representatives of the municipalities. It is better if this can be done within the same organization. The sick people's home is handled by the communes so we have to negotiate with all the communes in our area. So it is very difficult to go to a central organization to discuss these issues. In addition, not all the communes are alike, some handle their responsibilities very well and others do not.

Another clinic chief mentioned that,

All reforms demand a lot of work to build up the system in the beginning of the reform, and I think there has been too little effort in that. It was a big reform that was not anticipated and there are no doctors in the communes at the moment, but I think there should be more medical staffing in the communes. Because the patients are inhabitants of the old people's home and many of them have different diseases, it is a risk that they are not well-taken care of.

A cardiologist in one of the hospitals in the Skane region mentioned, in answer to a question about the impact of the elderly reform, stated that,

The reform has created a lot of problems. We have a big problem in this hospital, where we have a shortage of hospital beds. The big problem is not the number of beds but the people who are treated and need to go to the local municipalities but they cannot be transferred because they cannot find a place for them.

So they end up staying in the hospital, occupying hospital beds, which means we do not have places for other patients. It has not worked as well as I had hoped. There is a big problem and it is very bureaucratic to try to get the patient out of the hospital to one of the municipalities.

Another hospital physician in the Skane region, however, thought that the Adel Reform has worked to the benefit of the hospital. As he asserted,

Of course, once a patient is medically ready for discharge, we can use some pressure to discharge the patient to the municipalities. But I think there is a lack of doctors in that system and actually there is a law against employing doctors in that public system.

Privatization in Swedish Health Care

Since the introduction of so-called internal market reforms, Sweden, like other European countries has experimented with different health care payment administrative modalities with an eye towards further privatization in the health care system. Included in this model was the separation between health care purchasers and providers through the county councils, the introduction of a performance-based reimbursement DRG system, the privatization of St Goran's hospital and other hospitals in Stockholm and competition among hospital providers. This study was interested in exploring the perspectives of health care providers and health economists on the introduction of these reforms.

More specifically the respondents, even those in other cities were asked to assess the wider implication of the privatization of St Goran's Hospital in Stockholm and to assess whether such trends were likely to continue given the current health financing needs in Sweden. Ninety-five percent of the respondents reported that privatization within the Swedish health care system has been positive and long overdue. With the exception of only two hospital doctors, all the interviewed participants reported that the privatization of St. Goran's has been positive and encouraged future expansion of these benefits to other hospitals. But while most of the respondents saw the value in privatizing health care, most were quick to point out that such a policy should not cover university teaching hospitals. Ninety percent pointed to the benefit of having private and public hospitals side by side. They saw this as positive in forcing the public hospitals to become more efficient in the delivery of health care services. As one family care practitioner noted, "No, I do not think it is good to privatize every hospital but it is good to have both public and private hospitals."

In answer to the benefits of privatizing St. Goran's Hospital a chief of clinic mentioned that, " Yes, well, of course, I think many of the doctors who work there think it is good because they have their own possibilities to plan their education, but I think they focus too much on the money." Another health economist mentioned that, "a solution to health care costs is more privatization, but stressed that the current government had just passed a law prohibiting further privatization of hospitals in the health care system." Another hospital doctor replied, "Yes, I think more hospitals in Sweden should be privatized because it will be cost-effective to do so. My personal view is that the university hospitals should be state-owned and financed by the state, and smaller hospitals should be privatized because these hospitals now are not cost-effective." However, on the benefits of market reforms in the health care system, one hospital physician cautioned that,

> There is a danger to the health care system from privatization and that is not very good because it allows you to figure out how to make money with the least effort. For example, we have a lot of patients referred to us because we have a very specialized unit. The radiology services at the private units are not well done. I worked extra hours last year in an endoscopic unit downtown and it is obvious that you can make more money by doing unnecessary things and by examining healthy patients rather than sicker patients. There are so many examples of these and I think politicians should be in tune with these things but I am not sure they are.

From their responses, an overwhelming number of physicians were in favor of privatizing more of the health care system except at the teaching hospitals. Some also voiced concern that, while privatization will encourage efficiency and productivity, there is also the danger that privatization may undermine the equity and solidarity so ingrained in Swedish society and, inter alia, the Swedish health care system.

Care Guarantees

In the early 1990s, in an attempt to reduce the waiting time for patients, the Swedish government and the Federation of County Councils introduced care guarantees for some operations. In 2006, care guarantees was extended to cover all operations.

The respondents were asked their views on the previous and current policies on guarantees and whether they supported this expansion. The responses were mixed. About fifty percent of the respondents looked favorably on this legislation. As one private physician stated, "If I cannot take care of my patients within three months, then I am not fulfilling my responsibilities to my patients. So I think this is generally good for the patients."

However, a clinic chief felt this reform was too simplistic. In his elaboration, he indicated that

> [The care guarantee] is a political decision and it is very important for the politicians to be able to say that now we can guarantee that every patient can be taken care of within three months. However, this is very counter-productive because it does not allow for a reasonable handling of health priorities, since patients with minor and severe cases must be taken care off at the same time and certainly we do not have the resources to take care of them at the same time.

Another hospital urologist in response to a question about the care guarantee was felt that:

> [The care guarantee] is a joke and incredibly funny, because it does not relate to the diagnoses. If we have a patient with cancer, we cannot wait too long, but if we have a patient with a cold, he can wait, so this is really a political goal. Okay, I think it puts pressure on us working in the system, and we try to cope with that system. And if it fails, we have a benchmark to compare with. So it may not be so bad at all, but for many patients it is better for them to know when and where a certain procedure could be done and if you got a hip replacement and you got an appointment for December 10th, then it could be okay. But in many cases, you do not know when you will be operated on because of the care guarantee.

Working Conditions

On average, primary care and hospital physicians reported seeing between 15 to 20 patients every day. Heads of departments reported working an average of 45 hours a week. All the physicians interviewed were members of the Swedish Medical Association. All, with the exception of two hospital physicians, reported being satisfied with their work and willing to recommend their jobs to their immediate family members. This perspective appears unchanged since my last study in 2001 (Quaye, 2001).

A primary care physician in private practice stated that,

> In general, I am satisfied with my work. I have a very heavy load. Our days do not end until about 7 or 8 P.M. but actually it is very nice work and I think I get a lot of affection and confidence from my patients, which makes living worthwhile. But it is also very demanding and very hard. I will recommend the work to others but will insist that each family physician should not be responsible for more than fifteen hundred patients. This is because we have too many patients and this causes a lot of stress and dissatisfaction since one cannot possibly have the time to take care of the patients properly. That is why a case load of twelve hundred patients is ideal for a good doctor.

A private cardiologist stated that, "Yes, I must say that for the most part, I am satisfied with my work. I think I do not work too much. I think I have a very interesting job, and I feel I am able to cope with the work. One could always want more money, but I am generally satisfied with my work."

However, one emergency room physician in Southern Sweden commented that,

> We are getting less and less money through the hospital. The resources are just decreasing all the time. I am satisfied as a doctor but not satisfied with what I do for the patients. That is the reason why I am going to Denmark because in Denmark as a doctor you work with patients, but here you have a lot of administration and less patient care. I am constantly frustrated because I have no beds for patients. Today, we have no beds available for the patients and that is the greatest problem and that is the second reason that I want to leave.

A hospital physician in Malmo, in answer to a question about the relationship between the county council and the medical profession, had this to say,

> In general, we [doctors] like our job, but we do not like our employer. There are many reasons why, and one of them is that it is a little bit unclear if we should work more or less. If we work less, we get criticized because we produce too little, and if we work harder, we are criticized because we are expensive. It is not easy to find the exact, perfect amount of work.

Future of Health Care in Sweden

The last theme of this study explored the perspectives of health economists, Federation of County Council members and various types of physicians on the future of health care practice in Sweden. Several topics were explored. Four major future challenges were raised by the respondents: controlling health care costs, improving patient safety, elderly care and revisiting the Swedish solidarity principle.

The first topic identified was about controlling health care costs by introducing greater privatization in the health care system. As one clinic chief stated, "I think at the moment we have reached the limit with taxes so the challenge will be how to pay for the increased cost of health care and I do not know how we will resolve it. I think more privatization will be the answer, but the current government just passed the law prohibiting privatization of hospitals in the health care system." She added, "We have a lot of resources, but I do not think they are functioning well. One of the disturbing factors is the constant re-organization in the health care system [which] takes too long and takes too much time away from productivity and efficiency in the health care system."

A primary care physician in private practice noted, "We need better cooperation between the GPs and those at the hospitals. And something has to be done to the DRG system because it is not fair. I think they should give us more money or put more money into primary health care so we can take care of more patients."

A chief of clinic declared that :

> There is the need for improvement in patient security and safety. There are risks in health care that we should take care of and we need to find a system for that. One way to do so is to have better recording of outcomes of our activities and a follow-up of the DRG and to make it easier for the hospitals and the doctors to follow up on what is happening to the patient.

Another security issue mentioned as requiring immediate attention is psychiatric care. As one surgeon noted,

> We are closing down the big institutions and throwing people into the street and saying, you have to get along by yourself. This is a major challenge for the system. You know Swedish foreign minister Anna Lindh was killed by a person who in the same day [in 2003] had sought medical care at a psychiatric clinic and was denied access.

However, a health economist predicted that "the 'stop law' will be abolished and the idea of public financing of health care will not change, because there is a consensus on that. I foresee, though, an increase in the number of health care providers." From the perspective of a hospital surgeon, "The health care system is extremely dependent on the political majority and that is a problem if you have changes in the parties. I can live with either side having the majority but find it difficult with all these constant changes of direction in the health care system." One hospital cardiologist stated, " I hope that we can get some discussion about priorities to see what our responsibility in health care is. That needs to be addressed not only within the health care system but also by the politicians and the general public so that they know what is reasonable and expected from health care providers."

A third issue is the need to reform various special care situations, including elderly care by creating greater incentives for privatization and allowing greater collaboration between the county councils and the municipalities.

Fourth is the need to reconsider the Swedish solidarity principle in the face of the relatively high ratio between the working population and those dependent on the generosity of the welfare state. Several mentioned the need to address this problem, since the welfare state cannot support both the increasing number of Swedes who are on disability, sick leave or unemployed, and the aged given the fact that about eighteen percent of the Swedish population is 65 years and above and the number is rising. That is the Swedish challenge.

Discussion

This paper has examined the perspectives of hospital and private physicians, health economists, and Federation of County Council members on current trends within the Swedish health care system. The respondents generally believed that the basic structure of the Swedish health care system has remained intact and that the several reforms of the early 1990s introducing financial incentives into the health care system have worked well. The DRG system, though not popular among some health care providers, especially physicians seems to have worked for the purposes intended. The majority of Swedish physicians interviewed expressed some satisfaction with their work. A majority praised the internal reforms as contributing to rather stable health care expenditures, which are low compared with the United States and Canada. A majority of the respondents supported the care guarantee provisions even though some expressed reservation about its implementation without a careful review of priorities in the health care system.

Major issues raised consistently by the respondents included the need to carefully re-evaluate the allocation of responsibilities between the county council and the municipalities concerning care of the elderly. Others suggested that greater cooperation should exist among the county councils and the municipalities, and that the law should be changed to allow the municipalities to employ not only nurses but doctors as well. Overwhelmingly, the respondents believed that general practitioners should come to play a major role in health care, including the role of gatekeepers as in the Danish health care system.

Above all, a number voiced concern about the inability of the welfare state to continue to meet the health aspirations of all Swedes, given the high and growing dependency ratio in the population. Several decried the constant changes (every four year) in the Swedish health care in response to changes in government. From the perspectives of several clinic chiefs, these changes do not augur well for a well-planned Swedish health care system. Some clinic chiefs suggested that there should be greater centralization in health care planning and that the national government should play a much greater role in this.

Sweden has experimented with different health care modalities for the past twelve years. Yet, while these changes have altered to some extent the way in which health care is financed, the fundamentals of the welfare state and the solidarity principle, the hallmark of the Swedish experience, have remained virtually unchanged, an enduring social experiment. Sweden is leading the way in showing what governments can do in a global society where access to health care is of paramount importance. All Swedes can feel proud of a well-planned health care system.

Chapter Seven

Challenges for the Welfare States in Europe and the Way Forward

In this chapter I explore the challenges facing the health care in the welfare states of Europe. In a 1998 *New York Times* article, Craig Whitney stated that, "The high level of health care offered by the welfare states of Western Europe was long the envy of much of the rest of the world, but they can no longer afford the vast amounts required to pay for unlimited benefits" (p.1) That this is a truism can be seen in the various market-oriented reforms introduced in Western Europe to address mounting health care costs. After all, the proportion of Gross Domestic Product devoted to health care was already high even in the early 1980s: The United Kingdom devoted about 7.6 percent of GDP to health, Denmark, 8.6 percent, the Netherlands, 8.9 percent, Belgium, 9.0 percent, Sweden at 8.7 percent and Germany at 10.7 percent (Swedish Association of Local Authorities and Regions, 2005). At the same time, the number of citizens waiting for elective surgeries had increased and patients complained about their limited access to care and their dissatisfaction with the health care system

It was under such conditions that in 1989 a British White Paper on proposals for the National Health Service introduced among its major goals the need to encourage competition among health care providers through formation of hospital trusts with general practitioners as fund holders. About 20 percent of the total British National Health Service budget went directly to the fund holders, the equivalent of the United States health maintenance organizations (HMOs). Because of these measures, the primary care physicians had clear incentives to hold down medical costs by reducing over-treatment of patients. Since the financial payments to these physicians were partly tied to their ability to hold down cost, some have argued that such measures have led to further under-treatment of patients. In a nutshell, many British general practitioners have formed HMOs that then negotiate contracts with hospitals and surgeons. As a result, some 4,333 such hospitals trusts and about half the general practitioners in the U.K are directly involved in the delivery of care (Whitney, 1996:1).

Similarly, as alluded to earlier, the Dekker Reform in the Netherlands and the Blum Reform in Germany focused on the introduction of market-oriented systems in the delivery of health care. For example, to address problems with inefficiency and uncoordinated financing structures, the Dekker Reforms gave providers competitive incentives to produce cost-effective care, and also streamlined the private insurance sector by creating a common risk-related premium in an attempt to avoid the skimming of patients and the dumping of patients into the exceptional medical expense scheme. It also encouraged the most inefficient hospitals to close, and gave patients more health care choices (OECD, 1995).

Under the Blum Reform in Germany, competition among health care providers was encouraged through a DRG-based reimbursement payment system, and new regulations were introduced to monitor government-run sickness funds. There are over eight hundred and fifty sickness funds covering 92 percent of the German population. The private sector role in German health care is very small. Private insurance just covers eight percent of the population and only those with incomes over the maximum for signing up with a sickness fund (Whitney, 1996). Incentives were offered to reduce centralization of existing funds and the government imposed strict controls on health care costs. Another area of cost cutting was in drug prescriptions. Physicians had clear incentives not to over-prescribe and in some cases were held financially liable for doing so. In an attempt to reduce excess capacity in health care, the government actively pursued policies to reduce the number of physicians in active practice in Germany. These measures, together with increased patient's fees allowed the government to contain health care costs in Germany.

In France, a similar approach was taken. Apart from the use of clear incentives in its reimbursements to hospitals and physicians, the government aggressively limited certain services and required the purchase of supplementary health insurance for those services not covered under existing sickness funds. Unlike, in Sweden, French doctors are not state employees, and their bills are only 70 percent reimbursed by the health insurance that the government requires virtually everybody to subscribe to (Whitney, 1996). In addition, the government has pursued a tough prescription policy and increased user fees for patients. Through other financial incentives, the French government encouraged patients to use their general practitioners before consulting a specialist, thus strengthening the position of general practitioners as gate keepers in the French health delivery system.

In the same way, Sweden, despite reduced health care expenditures in the 1990s, recognized the inefficiencies within its system. Reforms introduced in Sweden included: free patient choice of doctors, privatization of one major hospital, the formation of hospital trusts, and the merger of specific teaching hospitals, especially in Stockholm County, and the introduction of care guarantee waiting time of three months or less as well as the introduction of a performance reimbursement system in health care.

As reported throughout this book, the Swedish experiment with financial incentives seemed to have worked very well. As reported by several studies, the introduction of the performance-based reimbursement payment system has led to increased productivity and efficiency in health care (Bergman, 1998; Hakansson, 1999; Forsberg, 2001; Quaye, 2001). As reported in my study and also confirmed by Forsberg (2001), performance-based reimbursement has been a useful way to create the right incentives in health care decisions. As she reported, in a study comparing Stockholm County (where 100 % of hospital budgets was based on performance-based reimbursement) with 10 other county councils without this payment system, "Physicians in Stockholm were more positively affected by financial incentives than their colleagues in the other ten counties (p.3). Forsberg (2001:17) observed that cost awareness was greater among physicians in Stockholm than in the other ten counties and that physicians in Stockholm more often discharged patients prematurely, feeling greater pressure to take patients out of intensive care units because of cost considerations.

Furthermore, Bruce and Jonsson compared productivity between "so-called" model counties and a set of "14 control counties" and concluded that the model counties increased their productivity more than the control counties. The productivity was 7%, 12.1%, 14.1%, 16% and 17.4% for the five model counties and these figures were achieved without a reduction in the quality of care nor any under-treatment, or insensitivity to the perverse incentives of DRG creep. On a much larger scale, the length of stay in hospitals decreased from an average of 11 days in 1970, to 7.9 days in 1992, to 6.1 days in 2002 (Swedish Association of Local Authorities and Regions, 2005).

The Swedish average length of hospital stay is shorter by 45 percent compared to that in France and Germany. Only Denmark and Finland have shorter average hospital stays. In a recent study, Swedish patient satisfaction ranked higher than in most European countries. About sixty percent of Swedes reported being satisfied with their health care. Only nine percent were dissatisfied with the health care delivery system.

Six major challenges facing the Swedish health care system are: the relatively untapped role of primary health care physicians; the need for rationing of health care, particularly when it comes to elective operations; high demands on the health care system because of virtually free access to health care; high cost of prescription drugs; an aging population (17 % of Swedes are over 65 years of age); and the delays in and greater use of hospital services.

As Swedes look-to the future, one thing is certain. The welfare state as we know it can no longer sustain the generous benefits that Swedes have traditionally enjoyed. Faced with mounting budget deficits, reluctance on the part of the national and county governments to raise taxes further to fund health care programs, and a rising dependent population, given the large numbers of Swedes who have taken early retirement or are on disability and or unemployed, the welfare system is reeling. As we look across the globe, Sweden is not alone. In Italy, France, and Germany, there are deep constraints on the welfare states' ability to meet its solidarity goals.

In my interviews with health economists and county politicians, it has become clear to me that a new way to finance the health care system is becoming increasingly likely. For a start, I think that Swedes are gradually moving into a two-tier health care system—basic health coverage for all, and additional supplementary insurance or contributions by those who are in a position to afford other care. What also seems likely is more privatization in the Swedish health care system. The success of St. Gorans Hospital as a private for-profit hospital has shown how effective health care can be delivered without compromising quality care. While the lessons from St. Goran's may not be ideal, it is clear that Sweden has no choice but to introduce more financial incentives in health care. It is becoming also increasing likely that patients will be asked to pay more and that Swedes with enough money will be encouraged to seek the more advanced medical help outside the county.

What is clear is that in the midst of these changes, the role of the primary care physician in the medical division of labor is uncertain. The Swedish government can endeavor to strengthen the position of the primary care physicians by allowing for greater privatization in the primary health care sector. This can be achieved through better conditions of work, reduction in the number of patients per general practitioner, and greater sensitization of Swedes to the important role play by primary care physicians. The position of general practitioners in the Danish health care system is a novelty and a lesson for Sweden. The Danes boast of a well-developed primary care sector because of its privatization. What the Danes have done is akin to the British system of fund holders and gate keeping of primary care physicians. Now is the time for Swedes to embrace this approach. In any case, the national government can play an active role in the restructuring of the entire Swedish health care system. Only this can forestall the danger of compromising and undermining the Health and Medical Services Act, which guarantees "good health care on equal terms for the entire population" (Glengard, Hjalte, Svensson, and Anell, 2004).

Appendix

Thank you for deciding to complete this survey. Your response is important to this study. Please be fair and honest as possible in your answers to these questions. Please place a "X" in the box next to what you feel is the best answer to each question.

DIRECTIONS

- Please check the box next to the answer that pertains to you.
- Please answer to the best of your ability.
- If you do not know the answer to a question, simply skip that question and continue answering the remaining questions.

1. Age: [ ] 25–35   [ ] 36–45   [ ] 46–55   [ ] 56–65   [ ] 66+

2. Sex: [ ] Male   [ ] Female

3. Type of Physician:
   [ ] Primary Care
   [ ] Specialist Which Specialty _____

4. How many years have you been practicing medicine?
   _____ years.

5. Is your income based on:
   [ ] Fee-For-Service
   [ ] Capitation
   [ ] Both
   [ ] Other

6. What percentage of your practice is HMO based?
    1. 1–10%
    2. 11–20%
    3. 21–30%
    4. 31–40%
    5. 41–50%
    6. 51–

7. Does your arrangement with managed care include some type of incentive in the form of a bonus?
    [ ] Yes
    [ ] No

8. If yes, what factors are used to calculate the bonus? Does it include the following:
    [ ] referral of patient to specialists
    [ ] use of laboratory
    [ ] prescription of drugs
    [ ] quality of care determined by audits
    [ ] patients' ratings of their satisfaction with the care they received
    other _____

9. What type of insurance do you accept?:
    (check as many as pertain to you)
    [ ] Private
    [ ] Corporate
    [ ] Medicaid
    [ ] Medicare
    [ ] Other   please list _____
    Why _____
    _____
    _____
    _____
    _____

10. Are you in favor of Managed Care?
    [ ] Yes
    [ ] No

11. What does Managed Care mean to you?
    _____
    _____
    _____
    _____

Please rate each item on a scale of 1–3 with 1 indicating that you do not experience such pressure, 2–indicating that you experience some pressure but that it did not compromise care 3–indicating that such pressure did compromise care.

12. Do you feel pressured from HMO's to limit referrals?
    1. [ ]
    2. [ ]
    3. [ ]

13. Are you pressured to see more patients per day?
    1. [ ]
    2. [ ]
    3. [ ]

14. Do you feel that such pressure compromise patient care?
    1. [ ]
    2. [ ]
    3. [ ]

15. Do you feel pressured from HMO's to limit referrals?
    1. [ ]
    2. [ ]
    3. [ ]

16. Are you pressured to see more patients per day?
    1. [ ]
    2. [ ]
    3. [ ]

17. Do you feel that such pressure compromise patient care?
    1. [ ]
    2. [ ]
    3. [ ]

18. What effects do you perceive to be the impact of managed care on the patient?
    _____
    _____
    _____

19. How much has the effect of managed care been discussed in your practice?
    [ ] Much
    [ ] Very Much
    [ ] Not Much
    [ ] Not At All

20. I am satisfied with my work (medical practice)
    [ ] Strongly Agree
    [ ] Agree
    [ ] Not Much
    [ ] Not At All

21. I will recommend this profession highly to my children or relatives?
    [ ] Strongly Agree
    [ ] Agree
    [ ] Not Much
    [ ] Not At All

22. As a result of changes in health care, are doctors losing control under a managed care system?
    [ ] Yes
    [ ] No

23. Does managed care decrease a physician's autonomy?
    [ ] Yes
    [ ] No

    Explain:
    _____
    _____
    _____
    _____

24. If so then how:
    [ ] Clinical Freedom
    [ ] Income
    [ ] Autonomy
    [ ] Quality of Care

25. Are some doctors "better off" with managed care?
    [ ] Yes
    [ ] No

26. What type of physician is better off with managed care?
    _____

27. If so then how:
    [ ] Clinical Freedom
    [ ] Income
    [ ] Autonomy
    [ ] Quality of Care

28. Do you feel that managed care could be the solution for America's 37 million uninsured citizens?
    [ ] Yes
    [ ] No

29. The net income from your practice is:
    [ ] 90–100,000
    [ ] 110,000–150,000
    [ ] 160,000–200,000
    [ ] 210,000

30. What are the racial characteristics of your patients. What percentage are
    [ ] White
    [ ] Black
    [ ] Asian
    [ ] Latino
    [ ] Amish
    [ ] Native Americans

    Please elaborate:
    _____
    _____
    _____
    _____
    _____

31. Do you support HMO's patient bill of right? (right for patients to sue their HMO's)
    [ ] Yes
    [ ] No

32. How best should the U.S.A. reduce health care cost and address the problem of the uninsured?

33. In 1997, Oregon State legalized physician-assisted suicide. Do you believe that the State of Ohio should pass such a law?
    [ ] Yes
    [ ] No

    Please elaborate:
    _____
    _____
    _____
    _____

Questionnaire to Swedish Physicians

1. What is your position at this hospital or clinic?
2. How long have you been practicing medicine?
3. What is the Stockholm model?
4. How are hospitals and physicians paid in Sweden?
5. Is the DRG system a good method for reimbursement for hospitals?
6. How conscious are you about cost saving measures?
7. What is the average length of stay in your hospital?
8. What is the national average?
9. Do you favor more privatization of hospitals in Sweden such as St. Gorans hospital?
10. Should the County Council encourage more privatization in health care?
11. Should general practitioners (GPs) play a major role in health care delivery system in Sweden?
12. On the average, how many hours do you work?
13. Are you satisfied with your working conditions?
14. Will you recommend this profession to your relative? Why or why not?
15. Have patients care suffered as a result of these market reforms?
16. Describe some of the major changes in the Swedish health care system as it relates to issues of cost and delivery of care
17. How do you assess the introduction of the Stockholm model on hospital performance?
18. What is the current status of the Family Doctors' Legislation?
19. What has changed in the health care delivery system since the Social Democratic Party took power in the early 2000s?
20. What has been the impact of the introduction of the DRG system on physicians' behavior?
21. How will you characterize the relationship between the national government, county councils and the medical profession?
22. What is the future of medical practice in Sweden?
23. Are Swedish physicians better off under a Conservative or Social Democratic government?

Bibliography

Aker, S. *The Right to Health*. Michigan: University Microfilms International, 1980.

Anderson, G., and J. Poullier. "Health Spending, Access and Outcomes: Trends in Industrialized Countries." *Health Affairs* 18, no.3 (1999):178–92.

Anderson, G. and I. Karlberg. "Integrated Care for the Elderly: The Background and Effects of the Reform of Swedish Care of the Elderly." *International Journal of Integrated Care* 1, no.1 (2000).

Anell, Anders. "The Monopolistic Integrated Model and Health Care Reform: The Swedish Experience." *Health Policy* 37 (1996): 19–33.

Averill, R. and Michael Kalison. "Structure of a DRG-Based Prospective Payment System." *DRGs: Their Design and Development*. Robert Fetter, David Brand and Dianne Gamache, eds. Ann Arbor, MI: Health Administration Press, 1991 (207–236).

Burfield, W., D. Hough, and W. Marder. "Location of Medical Education and Choice of Location of Practice." *Academic Medicine* 61 (1986): 545–554.

Bergman, Eric-Sven. "Swedish Models of Health Care Reform: A Review and Assessment." *International Journal of Health Planning and Management* 13 (1998): 91–106.

Berleen,G., S. Hakansson, C. Rehnberg, and G. Wennstrom. *The Reform of Health Care in Sweden: National Report to OECD*. Stockholm: SPRI, 1992.

Bodenheimer, T. and K. Sullivan. "How Large Employers Are Shaping the Health Care Market Place." *New England Journal of Medicine* 338 (1998): 1003–1007.

Bruce, A. and E. Jonsson. *Competition in the Provision of Health Care: The Experiences of US, Sweden and Britain*. Aldershot: Arena, 1996.

Bardsley, M., J. Coles, and L. Jenkins. *DRGs and Health Care: The Management of Case Mix*. London: King Edward's Hospital Fund for London, 1989.

Bjorkman, J. "Who Governs the Health Sector?" *Comparative Politics* (1985): 399–421.

Charpentier, C. and L. Samuelson. *Effekter av en sjukvardsreform: erfarenhter av Stockholmsmodden*. Sollentuna: Nerenius and Santerus Forlag, 1999.

Cohen, A., J. Cantor, D. Barker, and R. Hughes. "Young Physicians and the Future of the Medical Profession." *Health Affairs* 9 (1990): 138–148.

Cleary, P, and B. Landon. "A Conceptual Model of the Effects of Health Care Organizations on the Quality of Medical Care." *Journal of the American Medical Association* 279 (1998): 1377–1382.

Duran-Arenas, L. and M. Kennedy. "The Constitution of Physicians' Power: A Theoretical Framework for Comparative Analysis." *Social Science and Medicine* 32 (1991): 643–8.

Davis, K., G. Anderson, D. Rowland, and E. Steinberg. *Health Care Cost Containment*. Baltimore: The Johns Hopkins University Press, 1990.

Dietrich, A., E. Nelson, J. Kirk, M. Zubikoff, and G. O'Connor. "Do Primary Physicians Actually Manage Their Patients' Fee For Service Care?" *Journal of the American Medical Association* (1988).

Dobre. D., T. Custers, and N. Klazinga. " DRGs Crossing The Borders: A Systematic Analysis of the Transferability of Reported DRGs Experiences to the Hospital Context in Eastern European Countries." (Review Copy) 2003.

European Observatory on Health Care Systems. *Health Care Systems in Transition*. London: The Open Society, 2001.

Federation of Swedish County Councils. *Monitoring The European Health For All Strategy*. Stockholm: Federation of Swedish County Councils, 1994.

———. *Health Care Utilization and Resources in Sweden 1980–1992*. Stockholm: Modin Tryck, 1993.

Faffel, M., ed. *Comparative Health Systems: Descriptive Analysis of Fourteen National Health Systems*. University Park, PA: Pennsylvania State University Press, 1995.

Fetter, Robert. *DRGs-Their Design and Implementation*. Ann Arbor, MI: Health Administration Press, 1991.

Franks, P., P. Nutting, and C. Clancy. "Gatekeeping Revisited: Protecting Patients From Overtreatment." *New England Journal of Medicine* 6 (1991): 425–9.

Forsberg, E. *Do Financial Incentives Make a Difference?* Uppsala: Acta Universitatis Upsaliensis, 2001.

———. Personal Interview. August 1999.

Forsberg, E., R. Axelsson, and B. Arnetz. "Performance-Based Reimbursement in Health Care: Consequences for Physicians' Cost Awareness and Work Environment." *European Journal of Public Health* 12 (2002): 44–50.

———. "Effects of Performance-Based Reimbursement in Healthcare." *Scandinavian Journal of Public Health* 28 (2000): 102–110.

———. "Performance-Based Reimbursement in Health Care." *European Journal of Public Health* 12 (2002): 44–50.

Forsberg, E. and Calltorp, J. *Ekonimiska Incitament Och Medicinskt Handlandee Forsta Aret Av Stockholmsdellen (Economic Incentives on Physician Behaviour)* Huddinge: Samhallsmedicinska Enteten, 1993.

Fact Sheet on Sweden. *The Health Care System in Sweden*. Stockholm: The Swedish Institute, 1995.

Federation of Swedish County Councils. *Health Care Data in Focus*. Stockholm, (Landstingsforbundet), www.skl.se, 2004.

Frenk, J. and Luis-Duran-Arenas. "The Medical Profession and the State." *The Changing Medial Profession*. Frederic Hafferty and John McKinlay, eds. New York: Oxford University Press, 1993 (25–42).

Friedson, E. *Professional Dominance: The Social Structure of Medical Care*. New York: Atherton Press, 1970.

Fetter, R., D. Brand, and D. Gamache. *DRGs: Their Design and Development*. Ann Arbor, MI: Health Administration Press, 1991.

Freeborn, D. and C. Pope. *Promise and Performance in Managed Care*. Baltimore, MD: Johns Hopkins University Press, 1994.

Glennerster, H. and M. Matsaganis. "The English and Swedish Health Reforms." *International Journal of Health Services* 24, no.2 (1994): 231–51.

Garpenby, P. *The State and the Medical Profession: A Cross-National Comparison of the Health Policy Arena in the United Kingdom and Sweden 1945–1985*. Sweden: Linkoping Studies in Arts and Science, 1989.

Glenngard, A., F. Hjalte, M. Svensson, and Anders Anell. "Health Care Systems in Transition: Sweden." *European Observatory on Health Systems and Policies*. Viada Bankauskaite, ed. Sweden: The Swedish Institute for Health Economics, 2004.

Hakansson, S. "New Ways of Financing and Organizing Health Care in Sweden." *International Journal of Health Planning and Management* 9 (1994): 103–124.

———. "Experiences of DRGs in Sweden 1985–1999." Paper presented at the 15th annual meeting of the International Working Conference on Patient Classification Systems in Europe, Odense, Denmark, September 1999.

Hakansson, S. and S. Nordling. "Sweden." *Health Care and Reform In Industrialized Countries*. University Park, PA: Pennsylvania University Press, 1997.

Ham, C., R. Robinson, and M. Benzeval. *Health Check: Health Care Reforms in an International Context*. London: Kings' Fund Institute, 1990.

Haug, M.R. "The Erosion of Professional Authority: A Cross-Cultural Inquiry in the Case of the Physician." *Milbank Memorial Fund Quarterly* 54 (1976): 83–106.

———. "Computer Technology and the Obsolescence of the Concept of Profession." *Work and Technology*. Marie R. Haug and Jacques Dofny, eds. Beverly Hills, CA: Sage, 1977.

Hafferty, F. and John McKinlay. *The Changing Medical Profession: An International Perspective*. New York: Oxford University Press, 1993.

Hillman, A. L., M. Pauly, and J. Kerstein. "How Do Financial Incentives Affect Physicians' Clinical Decisions and the Financial Performance of Health Maintenance Organizations?" *New England Journal of Medicine* 321 (1989): 86–92.

Hemenway, D., A. Killen, and S.B. Cashman. "Physicians' Responses to Financial Incentives: Evidence from a For-Profit Ambulatory Care Center." *New England Journal of Medicine* 322 (1990): 1059–63.

Iglehart, J. "The American Health Care System." *The New England Journal of Medicine* 340, no.1 (1999): 70–76.

Jonsson, E. "Has Reimbursement Per Patient Given More Value for Money?" Stockholm: Stockholm University, 1996.

Krause, E. *Death of the Guilds*. New Haven: Yale University Press, 1996.

MacDonald, R. "HMO Game." *Time* Magazine, 13 July, 1998.

McKinlay, J. and J. Stoeckle. "Corporatization and the Social Transforming of Doctoring." *International Journal of Health Services* 18 (1989): 191–205.

Marquis, J. " Physicians Seek Remedy." *Akron Beacon Journal* 7 March, (1999): B1.

Melden, M. "Medicaid and Managed Care." *Beyond Crisis.* Nancy McKenzie, ed. New York: Meridian Group, 1994.

Mosher, Steven. *The Right to Health: A Comparative Study of the Health Care Systems of the United States, Sweden, and Cuba.* Ann Arbor, MI: University Microfilm International, 1980.

Neuhauser, D. "Stimulating Cost-Effective Behaviour in Hospitals." *Health Policy* 7 (1987): 205–213.

O'Connor, S. and Joyce Lanning. "The End of Autonomy? Reflections on the Post-Professional Physician." *Health Care Management Review* 17, no.1 (1992): 63–72.

Organization for Economic Cooperation and Development (OECD). *Internal Markets in the Making.* Paris:OECD, 1995.

Quaye, R. "Struggle for Control: General Practitioners in the Swedish Health Care System." *European Journal of Public Health* 7 (1997): 248–53.

———. "Internal Market Systems in Sweden: Seven Years After the Stockholm Model." *European Journal of Public Health* 11 (2001): 380–385.

———. "Professional Integrity in the Age of Managed Care: Views of Physicians." *International Journal of Health Care Quality Assurance* 14, no.2 (2001): 82–86.

———. "Assessing the Impact of Cost Control Strategies on Swedish Physicians' Practice Behaviour." *International Journal of Health Care Quality Assurance* 16, no.5 (2003): 257–260.

Saltman, R, B. *Patient Choice and Patient Empowerment: A Conceptual Analysis.* Stockholm: Swedish Center for Business and Policy Studies, 1992.

———. "Recent Health Policy Initiatives in Nordic Countries." *Health Care Financing Review* 13, no.4 (1993): 157–66.

———. *Implementing Planned Markets in Health Care.* Philadelphia: Open University Press, 1995.

Starr, Paul. *The Social Transformation of American Medicine: The Rise of a Sovereign Profession and the Making of a Vast Industry.* New York: Basic Books, 1982.

Steinberg, A. *The Insider's Guide to HMOs.* New York: Plume Books, 1997.

Shortell, S. "Physicians as Double Agents: Maintaining Trust in an Era of Multiple Accountabilities." *Journal of the American Medical Association.* 280, no.2 (1998): 1102–1108.

Simon, S., R. Pan, A. Sullivan, N. Clark-Chiarelli, M. Connelly, and A. Peters. "Views of Managed Care–A Survey of Students, Residents, Faculty and Deans at Medical Schools in the United States." *The New England Journal of Medicine* 340, no.8 (1999): 959–961.

Svensson, H. and L. Garelius. *Have Economic Incentives Influenced the Decisions of Physicians?* Stockholm (Stencil): SPRI, 1994.

Swedish Association of Local Authorities and Regions. *Swedish Health Care in an International Context.* Stockholm: Alfa Print AB, 2005.

Serden, L. and Rikard Lindqvist. "Have the Introduction of DRG-Based Prospective Payment Systems Affected the Number of Diagnoses in Health Care Administrative Data?" Paper presented at the 17th PCS/E Conference, Bruges, Belgium, 10–13 October 2001.

Taira, Frances and Taira Deborah. "Patient 'Dumping' of Poor Families." *Families in Society* (1991): 409–15.

Warren, M., R. Weitz., and S. Kulis. "Physician Satisfaction in a Changing Health Care Environment." *Journal of Health and Social Behavior* 39 (1998): 357–67.

——. "The Impact of Managed Care on Physicians." *Health Care Management Review* 24, no.2 (1999): 44–56.

Weber, M. "Bureaucracy in From Max Weber." *Essays in Sociology*. H. Gerth and C.W. Mills, eds. New York: Oxford University Press, 1946.

Wolinsky, F. D. "The Professional Dominance Perspective, Revisited." *Milbank Quarterly* 66, no.2 (1988): 33–47.

Whitney, C. "Rising Health Costs Threaten Generous Benefits in Europe." *New York Times*, 5 August 1996.

Index

Adel reform, 6, 25, 26, 53–56
administrative work, 14–15, 51
Aker, S., 73
American Medical Association: Physician Masterfile, 18
Anderson, G., 73–74
Anell, Anders, 2, 6, 66, 73, 75
Arnetz, B., 39, 74
Averill, Richard, 36–37, 73
Axelsson, R., 39, 74

Bankkauskaite, V., 2
Bardsley, M., 36, 73
Barker, D., 74
Belgium, 63
Benzeval, M., 4, 75
Bergman, Eric-Sven, 5–6, 25, 26, 65, 73
Berleen, G., 1, 73
Bjorkman, J., 1, 2, 73
Blum Reform, vii, viii, 64
Bodenheimer, T., 12, 73
Bohus county: payment models, 5; purchaser organization, 5
Bohuslan county: productivity issues, 26
Brand, D., 75
Bruce, A., 26–27, 65, 73
Burfield, W., 21, 73

California: patient bill of rights, 18
Calltorp, J., 74
cancer, 25
Cantor, J., 74
"care guarantee," 26, 57–58
Cashman, S. B., 75
cataracts, 25
Center of Patient Classification System, 38
The Changing Medical Profession: An International Perspective (Hafferty and McKinlay), 75
The Changing Medical Profession (Frank and Luis-Duran-Arenas), 75
Charpentier, C., 27, 73
Cigna Directory of Physicians, 13
Clancy, C., 41, 74
Clark-Chiarelli, N., 76
Cleary, P., ix, 74
Cohen, A., 22, 74
Coles, J., 36, 38, 73
communication issues, 18
Comparative Health Systems: Descriptive Analysis of Fourteen National Health Systems (Faffel), 74
Connelly, M., 76
Conservative party (Sweden), 5, 34
Coronary surgery, 25

corporatism, definition of, 10
cost containment, 13. *See also* diagnostic-related groups (DRGs)
county councils (Sweden), 2, 4, 5–6, 6, 25, 55, 56, 57, 61, 74
cream-skimming patients, 27
Custers, T., 74

Dagmar Reform, 10
Dalara county, 52; payment models, 5; productivity issues, 26; purchaser organization, 5
Davis, K., 41, 74
"de-professionalization" of medical profession, ix; definition of, 10–11
Death of the Guilds (Krause), 75
decision making, 1, 15, 33, 50–53
Dekker Reform, vii, 64
Denmark, 4, 61, 63, 66
diagnosis accuracy, 51
diagnostic-related groups (DRGs), vii, 61; administration, 51; cheating, 52; costs, 51; data bases, 38; health economists and, 50–53; international comparisons, 37–38; length of hospital stay, 39; in Medicare, 36–37; outliers, 37, 38; as payment model, 5; quality of care, 39; reforms in Sweden, 25–29, 38–47; reimbursement payment system, viii; secondary diagnoses, 38–39; Stockholm Model, 25–29; Swedish physician attitudes toward, 39–47
Dietrich, A., 74
Do Financial Incentives Make a Difference? (Forsberg), 74
Dobre, D., 74
DRG creep, 27, 50–53, 51
DRGs. *See* diagnostic-related groups (DRGs)
DRGs-Their Design and Implementation (Fetter), 74
Duran-Arenas, L., 8–9, 74, 75

economic incentives, v; impact on medical profession, v, viii; performance-based reimbursement, v. *See also* diagnostic-related groups (DRGs)
Economic Incentives on Physician Behavior (Forsberg and Calltorp), 74
Effekter av en sjukvardsreform: erfarenhter av Stockholmsmodden (Charpentier and Samuelson), 73
elderly care, 6, 25, 26, 53–56, 60, 66
equity principle, 4, 9, 40
European Observatory on Health Care Systems, 2, 74

Fact Sheet on Sweden, 2, 74
Family Doctor's Legislation, 25, 26, 30–33
Federation of Swedish County Councils. *See* county councils (Sweden)
fee-for-service, 2, 7, 10, 12, 22, 26; quality of care, 22, 39; retrospective *vs.* prospective, 21
Fetter, Robert, 36–37, 74–75
financial incentives to limit care, 14, 40, 43–44, 50–53
Finland, 4
Forsberg, E., viii, 29, 39–41, 44, 46, 49, 65, 74
France, 64, 66
Franks, P., 41, 74
Freeborn, D., 12–13, 75
Frenk, J., 8–9, 75
Friedson, E., 8–10, 24, 75

Gamache, D., 75
Garelius, L., 27, 76
Garpenby, P., 2, 9–10
gatekeeping, 4, 7, 31, 32, 61
Gavelin, 38
gender issues, 24
Georgia, patient bill of rights, 18
geriatric care. *See* elderly care
Germany, 63, 66; Blum Reform, vii, viii, 64; centralization *vs.* pluralization, 9
Glennerster, H., 25–26, 75

Index

Glenngard, A., 2, 66, 75
Goteborg, Sweden, 51
Gothenburg, Sweden, data bases, 38

Hafferty, Frederic, 75
Hakansson, S., viii, 1, 3–4, 25–27, 38, 40–41, 65, 73, 75
Ham, C., 75
Haug, M. R., 8, 10–11, 75
Have Economic Incentives Influenced the Decisions of Physicians? (Svensson and Garelius), 76
Health and Medical Services Act (Sweden), 1, 66
health care: costs, 50, 51; future trends, 59–61; market-oriented systems, v–vii, 10, 12–24 (*see also* diagnostic-related groups (DRGs); rationing, 65; two-tier system, 66. *See also* Swedish health system
Health Care Cost Containment (Davis, Anderson, Rowland and Steinberg), 74
Health Care Data in Focus (Federation of Swedish Country Councils), 74
The Health Care System in Sweden (Fact Sheet on Sweden), 74
Health Care Systems in Transition (European Observatory on Health Care Systems), 74
Health Care Utilization and Resources in Sweden 1980-1992 (Federation of Swedish County Councils), 74
health economists, 50–53, 53, 60
health maintenance organizations (HMOs), 12–24, 17; HMO bill of rights, 18; study, 13–14
Health Systems Management Group (Yale University), 38
Hemenway, D., viii, 75
Hillman, A. L., viii, 41, 50, 75
hip replacement, 25
Hjalte, F., 2, 66, 75
HMO bill of rights, 18

hospitals, 2; length of hospital stay, 39, 65; productivity issues, 26; public *vs.* private, 56–57
Hough, D., 73
"house doctor scheme," 6
housing, 6, 26
Hughes, R., 74

Iglehart, J., 10, 12, 38, 75
infant mortality, 4
The Insider's Guide to HMOs (Steinberg), 76
insurance companies: clearinghouse, 18; practicing medicine without a license, 14
Italy, 66

Jenkins, L., 36, 38, 73
job satisfaction, 16–17, 22, 28, 31–33, 58–59; definition of, 24; DRGs and, 41, 45–46
Jonsson, E., 26–27, 65, 73, 75

Kaiser Permanante, 18
Kalison, Michael, 36–37, 73
Karlberg, I., 73
Kennedy, M., 74
Kerstein, J., 75
Killen, A., 75
Kirk, J., 74
Klazinga, N., 74
Krause, E., 8, 24, 75
Kulis, S., 12, 77

Landon, B., ix, 74
Lanning, Joyce, 10, 76
life expectancy, 4
Lindqvist, Rikard, 38–39, 76
Luis-Duran-Arenas, 75
Lund University hospital, 49

MacDonald, R., 13, 75
Malmo university hospital, 49, 59
managed care plans, 10, 12–24; cost containment, 13; definitions, 12–13,

14–15; quality of care, 22, 39; training in dealing with, 23
Marder, W., 73
Marquis, J., 13, 17, 76
Matsaganis, M., 26, 75
McKinlay, John, ix, 8, 10–11, 75–76
medical health care boards: as clearinghouse, 18
Medical Products Agency, 2
Medicare: prospective payment system, 36–37; retrospective payment system, 36–37
Melden, M., 17, 76
Ministry of Health and Social Affairs, 2
Monitoring the European Health for All Strategy (Federation of Swedish County Councils), 74
Mosher, Steven, 1–2, 76
municipality responsibility, 6, 25, 53–56, 60

National Board of Health and Welfare (Sweden), 2, 9, 30, 51
Nelson, E., 74
Netherlands, 63; Dekker Reform, vii, 64
Neuhauser, D., viii, 76
Nilsson, Carl-Axel, 38
Nordling, S., 3–4, 75
Nutting, P., 41, 74

O'Connor, G., 74
O'Connor, Stephen, 10, 76
Ohio: American Medical Association Physician Masterfile, 18; managed care, 12–24; medical profession in, viii; study of physicians and HMOs, 13–14, 18–22
Orebro county: productivity issues, 26
Organization for Economic Cooperation and Development (OECD), 1, 76
outliers, 37, 38

Pan, R., 76
Parsons, 8

A Patient Choice and Patient Empowerment: Conceptual Analysis (Saltman), 76
patients: "care guarantee," 26, 57–58; choice and, 15; HMO bill of rights, 18; overtreatment, 27; patient bill of rights, 18; underutilization of health systems, 50; waiting times, 25
Pauly, M., 75
payment methods: capitation, 22, 26; fee-for-service, 2, 7, 10, 12, 22, 26, 39; Medicare, 36–37; quality of care, 22, 39
Peters, A., 76
physicians: administrative work, 14–15; attitudes toward DRGs, 39–47; behavior, viii–ix, 40; choice and, 5, 15; cross-national comparison, 7–11; as double agents, 14; economic incentives' impact on, v, viii; job satisfaction, 16–17, 22, 24, 28, 31–33, 41, 45–46, 58–59; managed care and, viii, 39–47; primary care, 21–22, 23, 26, 30–33; professional autonomy, 16, 24, 28, 45–46; relations between specialists and primary care, 28, 30–31; salaries, 32; socialization of physicians, 7; specialties, 21–22, 23; training and practice locations, 21; U.S. compared to Swedish, viii; views on reforms, 28–29
planned market models of health care, 6
political parties, 7, 26, 34. *See also specific parties*
politics, 7, 26, 34
Pope, C., 12–13, 75
Poullier, J., 73
prescription drugs, 66
primary care physicians, 21–22, 23, 26, 30–33, 66; relations between specialists and primary care, 28, 30–31; working conditions, 31–33, 58–59

privatization, 5, 7, 33, 56–57, 66; family medicine, 30–33; Saint Goran's hospital, 33, 34
productivity issues, 4, 25, 26, 44, 65
profession, definition of, 8
professional autonomy, 16, 24, 28, 45-46. *See also* job satisfaction
The Professional Dominance: Social Structure of Medical Care (Friedson), 75
Promise and Performance in Managed Care (Freeborn and Pope), 75
Proposition 1992/93:160, 6
psychiatric care, 60
public control as value, 40, 60

quality of care, 22, 23, 39; "care guarantee," 26, 57–58; payment methods, 22, 39
Quaye, Randolph K., viii, 6, 10, 25–26, 30, 40, 48–49, 58, 65, 76

race issues, 24
referrals, 4, 15
Rehnberg, C., 1, 73
research methodology (Ohio studies): analysis, 19; drawbacks, 24; follow-up study, 18–22; initial study, 13–14; Likert scale, 13, 21, 22; questionnaires, 14, 18–19; respondents, 20; results, 14, 19–22; surveys, 13; training and practice locations, 21
research methodology (Swedish studies), 27–30, 40–47, 49–62; data analysis, 42; data collection, 28, 43; follow-up study, 49–62; limitations of study, 47; purpose, 40–41; questionnaires, 72; respondents, 43; results, 42–43, 50–61; study of DRGs, 28–29, 40–47; study of Stockholm Model, 27–30; surveys, 67–71
The Right to Health: A Comparative Study of the Health Care Systems of the United States, Sweden, and Cuba (Mosher), 76
The Right to Health (Aker), 73
Robinson, R., 4, 75
Rowland, D., 74

Saint Goran's hospital, 33, 34, 56, 66
Saltman, R. B., 4, 6, 40, 76
Samuelson, L., 27, 73
Serden, L., 38–39, 76
service integration, 4
Seven Crowns Reform, 2, 9
Shortell, S., 10, 13, 76
Simon, S., 12, 17, 76
Skane region (Sweden), 51
Social Democrat party (Sweden), 7, 26, 28, 34
social justice as social value, 4, 40
The Social Transformation of American Medicine, The: Rise of a Sovereign Profession and the Making of a Vast Industry (Starr), 76
solidarity principle, 9, 40, 60
Sormland county: payment models, 5; productivity issues, 26; purchaser organization, 5
specialist physicians, 28, 30–31, 45
Starr, Paul, 10, 76
state: authority of, 8; centralization *vs.* pluralization, 9; definition of, 8–10
Steinberg, A., 12, 17, 18, 41, 76
Steinberg, E., 74
Stockholm county. *See* Stockholm Model
Stockholm Model, 7, 25–29, 49, 51; data bases, 38; DRG points system, 25–29; maximum price list, 25; payment models, 5; performance-based reimbursement, v; productivity issues, 25–26; purchaser organization, 5
Stoeckle, J., ix, 10–11, 76
"stop law," 60

studies. *See* research methodology (Ohio studies); research methodology (Swedish studies)
Sullivan, A., 76
Sullivan, K., 73
surveys, 13, 67–71
Svensson, H., 2, 27, 66, 76
Svensson, M., 75
Sweden, 63; centalization *vs.* pluralization, 9
Swedish Association of Local Authorities and Regions, 2, 4, 76
Swedish Council of Technology Assessment in Health Care, 2
Swedish health reforms: Adel reform, 6, 25, 26, 53–56; "care guarantee," 26; choice, 4, 5, 25; diagnostic-related groups (DRGs), 36–47; efficiency incentives, 4, 5, 44; elderly care, 6, 25, 26; gatekeeping, 4; market systems and, 25–35; payment models, 5; productivity issues, 4, 26, 44; recruitment of practitioners, 4; referrals, 4; in the 1990s, 4–6; service integration, 4; utilization, 4; waiting times, 4, 28
Swedish health system, 5; centralization of system, 1, 33, 61; collective responsibility and, 1; competition, 5; current trends, 48–62; decentralization of decision making, 1, 33; expenditures, 1–2; financing flows, 3; funding of, 2; future trends, 59–61; hospitals, 2, 56-57, 65; inefficiencies in, viii, 25, 26, 44; medical profession in, viii, 25; natural law and, 1; number of facilities, 2; outpatient service uniform fee, 3; physician behavior, viii–ix; primary care use, 4, 26; private sector, 3, 4; privatization, 5; regionalization, 2; shared need and, 1; social justice and, 1; statistics, 4; types of care, 2; waiting lists, 25, 28
Swedish Medical Association, 9, 10, 58; journal, 38
Swedish Medical Board of Health and Welfare, 18
Swedish Medical Health Care Act, 34. *See also* Swedish health reforms
Swedish Medical Services Act, 9
Swedish Planning and Rationalizing Institute (SPRI), 38

Taira, Deborah, 41, 77
Taira, Frances, 41, 77
Tax Equity and Fiscal Responsibility Act of 1982 (TEFRA), 36
Texas: patient bill of rights, 18
theoretical concepts, 7–11
trade unions, 10

underutilization of health systems, 50
United Kingdom, 63–64
United States: managed care, 12–24; medicare, 36–37
urinary infection, 51

Varde, 26
Vastra-Gotland region (Sweden), 51

Warren, M., 12, 17, 77
Weber, M., 8, 77
Weitz, R., 12, 77
welfare state, 7; European challenges, 63–66; health care as component of, 1; market reforms and, v, 48–62; *vs.* private finance, viii, 48–62
Wennstrom, G., 1, 73
Whitehead, 26
Whitney, Craig, 63–64, 77
Wolinsky, F. D., 11, 77

Zubikoff, M., 74

Made in the USA
Monee, IL
28 April 2026